THE MAUDSLEY
The Maudsley Series

THE MAUDSLEY SERIES

HENRY MAUDSLEY, from whom the series of monographs takes its name, was the founder of The Maudsley Hospital and the most prominent English psychiatrist of his generation. The Maudsley Hospital was united with the Bethlem Royal Hospital in 1948 and its medical school, renamed the Institute of Psychiatry at the same time, became a constituent part of the British Postgraduate Medical Federation. It is now a school of King's College, London, and entrusted with the duty of advancing psychiatry by teaching and research. The South London & Maudsley NHS Trust, together with the Institute of Psychiatry, are jointly known as The Maudsley.

The monograph series reports high quality empirical work on a single topic of relevance to mental health, carried out at the Maudsley. This can be by single or multiple authors. Some of the monographs are directly concerned with clinical problems; others are in scientific fields of direct or indirect relevance to mental health and that are cultivated for the furtherance of psychiatry.

Editor
Professor A. S. David MPhil MSc FRCP MRCPsych MD

Assistant Editor
Professor T. Wykes BSc PhD MPhil

The Maudsley Series

The Extremes of the Bell Curve

Excellent and Poor School Performance and Risk for Severe Mental Disorders

James H. MacCabe

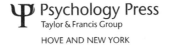

Psychology Press
Taylor & Francis Group
HOVE AND NEW YORK

First published 2010
by Psychology Press
27 Church Road, Hove, East Sussex BN3 2FA

Simultaneously published in the USA and Canada
by Psychology Press
270 Madison Avenue, New York, NY 10016

Psychology Press is an imprint of the Taylor & Francis Group, an Informa business

Copyright © 2010 Psychology Press

Typeset in Times by Garfield Morgan, Swansea, West Glamorgan
Printed and bound in Great Britain by TJ International Ltd,
Padstow, Cornwall
Cover design by Lisa Dynan

This publication has been produced with paper manufactured to
strict environmental standards and with pulp derived from
sustainable forests.

British Library Cataloguing in Publication Data
A catalogue record for this book is available from the British Library

Library of Congress Cataloging-in-Publication Data
    MacCabe, James.
    The extremes of the bell curve : excellent and poor school
performance and risk for severe mental disorders / James Hunter
MacCabe.
        p. cm.
    Includes bibliographical references and index.
    ISBN 978-1-84872-045-9 (hardback)
    1. Academic achievement–Psychological aspects–Sweden. 2.
Mental illness–Etiology. I. Title.
    LB1062.6.M33 2010
    370.15'2–dc22

                                                2009042487

ISBN: 978-1-84872-045-9 (hbk)

ISSN: 0076-5465

Contents

List of figures

List of tables

Preface

This book is a detailed description of the rationale, methods and results of the Study of Premorbid School Performance in Schizophrenia and other Psychoses (SP₃), which I conducted between 2004 and 2007, in collaboration with colleagues in Stockholm and London. At the time of writing I believe it remains the largest study to date to investigate the association between school performance in childhood and risk for psychosis in adulthood.

The term 'bell curve' refers to the shape of the distribution of IQ scores, or school grades, in the population. The notion of the bell curve was made famous (or infamous) by Hernstein and Murray, in their 1994 book of the same name (Herrnstein and Murray, 1994). The central finding of this research is that individuals at the highest and lowest ends of the bell-shaped distribution of school grades are at increased risk of severe mental disorders, compared with those with intermediate scores. I should make it clear that this book does not have any bearing on the controversial claims made in Herrnstein and Murray's book, particularly about alleged ethnic IQ differences.

I have tried to make the research accessible to a broader audience, such as other mental health professionals, educationalists, people suffering from psychoses, their families, or anyone else who may be interested in this work. To that end, I have tried to use as few technical terms as possible, and to define those that may be unfamiliar to non-specialists. The first three chapters are particularly aimed at this audience, and provide an introduction to the epidemiology of psychosis, with particular emphasis on cognitive performance and creativity.

The remainder of the book describes in detail the methods of the study itself, the results, and a discussion of the findings. I hope that this part of the book will be of interest to schizophrenia researchers and epidemiologists, and will provide a complete record of the study, warts and all, of the kind that is never possible within the constrained word limits of academic journals. To this end, I have included a level of detail that some will inevitably prefer to skim over. As far as possible, and particularly in the results section, I have placed many of the tables in an appendix, and ended each section with a brief summary, so that those who do not wish to wade through the finer detail can nevertheless follow the gist of the material. I have also tried to maintain a narrative style, spelling out in detail my reasoning for the decisions along the way, from study design through to analysis.

The line between readability and precision is not always an easy one to tread, and some will find my language too formal and pedantic, whereas others will berate my casual and imprecise style. If I upset roughly equal numbers of people in both camps then I will have succeeded.

I hope it goes without saying that my use of the masculine personal pronoun 'he' rather than 'he/she' and other clumsy alternatives is for the sake of readability and is not designed to exclude females or to cause offence.

James MacCabe
June 2009

Acknowledgements

With apologies to Oscar Wilde, to be supervised by one of the world's leading experts in one's chosen field may be regarded as good fortune, but two looks a bit like overindulgence. Robin Murray and Tony David, who supervised the PhD on which this work is based, have indulged me not only with their intellectual input, but also with patience, tolerance and humour. I am deeply indebted to them both.

My warmest thanks also to my colleagues at the Department of Medical Epidemiology and Biostatistics at Karolinska Institutet: Mats Lambe, Sven Cnattingius, Camilla Björk, and especially Christina Hultman. I would like to thank the Medical Research Council and Department of Health, who jointly funded my training fellowship which funded this research.

CHAPTER ONE

Background

WHAT IS SCHIZOPHRENIA?

Definition

The term *schizophrenia* was coined by Eugen Bleuler in the early twentieth century, and is derived, somewhat unhelpfully, from the Greek *schizo-* ($\Sigma\chi\iota\zeta$o = split/divide), and *phrenos* ($\varphi\rho\varepsilon\nu\acute{o}\varsigma$ = mind). Perhaps owing to this etymology, the words 'schizophrenia', and especially 'schizophrenic', have acquired a completely unrelated colloquial usage, whereby they are used to refer to a paradox or contradiction. More troublingly, many people hold the erroneous belief that people with schizophrenia have a 'split personality' or are subject to sudden dangerous transformations from normality to madness, similar to the character of Dr Jekyll and his alter-ego Mr Hyde, in the Victorian novella by Robert Louis Stevenson (Stevenson, 1886).

The modern concept of schizophrenia is based on Emil Kraepelin's descriptions of *dementia praecox*, which in turn drew on previous accounts by Haslam, Morel, Pinel and others (Adityanjee et al., 1999). Schizophrenia is a severe and chronic mental disorder, which usually manifests itself in early adulthood, and is characterised by a disparate range of symptoms, which despite their superficial unconnectedness, frequently co-occur in the same individual.

The most obvious symptoms to most observers are the so-called positive symptoms. Hallucinations (perceptions without an external source) occur in

1

almost all cases. These include auditory hallucinations (primarily hearing voices), although hallucinations are sometimes also experienced in other sensory domains, such as touch or smell. A second feature that is almost universal is the presence of delusions (fixed, false beliefs, which are out of keeping with the person's cultural background), and these are commonly paranoid or persecutory in content. Disorganised and erratic behaviour is frequent, as is thought disorder (severely disjointed or tangential connections between thoughts, and idiosyncratic vocabulary and grammar, manifesting as speech that is difficult to follow or even unintelligible). Over time, and often beginning before the onset of the positive symptoms described above, there is, in most cases, a marked deterioration in occupational and social functioning, often described as 'negative symptoms'.

Is schizophrenia a valid concept?

There has been fierce debate for over a century as to whether schizophrenia exists at all, whether it constitutes a single disorder or a collection of disorders, to what extent it can be demarcated from other disorders, and whether it is separable from normal functioning categorically, or only by degree. At the heart of all these debates lies the fundamental question of what defines a disease, and the uncomfortable truth that the causes and neurobiological basis of schizophrenia remain obscure.

Although there is clear evidence from many fields of research, including genetics, pharmacology, neuroimaging and epidemiology, that patients with schizophrenia differ on average from the remainder of the population, there is not, and may never be, an unambiguous biological 'test' that can reliably differentiate between people with a diagnosis of schizophrenia and healthy individuals. Instead, the diagnosis of schizophrenia is based on signs and symptoms. Signs are the clinician's observations of the appearance, behaviour or speech of the patient (such as 'this patient appears to be responding to hallucinations'). Symptoms are experiences volunteered by the patient, (such as 'I can hear a voice echoing my thoughts'). In fact, it is more accurate to say that symptoms are the diagnostician's evaluation of the patient's own account of his/her perceptions, experiences and beliefs. Thus, schizophrenia, like most psychiatric 'diagnoses', is more accurately described as a syndrome (a group of signs and symptoms that frequently co-occur) than a disease. It is also important to note that the assessment of signs and symptoms involves many subjective judgements on the part of the diagnostician, and often also on the part of the patient.

Scientific definition

The subjective nature of psychiatric diagnosis was highlighted by the anti-psychiatry movement in the 1960s and 1970s, and became a source of embarrassment to psychiatrists. Furthermore, it became clear that research efforts in identifying causes and treatments for mental disorders were being hindered by lack of consistency in the way that these disorders were defined. The response to this problem was to develop formal diagnostic criteria for mental disorders, which would be as objective and reliable as possible.

There are currently two dominant standards in Western psychiatry for the classification of psychiatric disorders: the *International Classification of Disease*, currently in its tenth edition (ICD–10), administered by the World Health Organization (WHO, 1992), and the *Diagnostic and Statistical Manual of Mental Disorders*, currently in its fourth edition (DSM–IV), published by the American Psychiatric Association (APA, 1994).

ICD–10 defines schizophrenia as follows:

> The schizophrenic disorders are characterized in general by fundamental and characteristic distortions of thinking and perception, and affects that are inappropriate or blunted. Clear consciousness and intellectual capacity are usually maintained although certain cognitive deficits may evolve in the course of time. The most important psychopathological phenomena include thought echo; thought insertion or withdrawal; thought broadcasting; delusional perception and delusions of control; influence or passivity; hallucinatory voices commenting or discussing the patient in the third person; thought disorders and negative symptoms.
>
> The course of schizophrenic disorders can be either continuous, or episodic with progressive or stable deficit, or there can be one or more episodes with complete or incomplete remission. The diagnosis of schizophrenia should not be made in the presence of extensive depressive or manic symptoms unless it is clear that schizophrenic symptoms antedate the affective disturbance. Nor should schizophrenia be diagnosed in the presence of overt brain disease or during states of drug intoxication or withdrawal.
>
> (WHO, 1992)

This is followed by more specific diagnostic criteria for the various subtypes of schizophrenia.

The existence of these subtypes reveals another aspect of schizophrenia that dogs research efforts: its clinical heterogeneity, or variability. Two individuals with no overlap in their symptoms might both be diagnosed with schizophrenia, whereas another patient may suffer from auditory hallucinations at one time, then apathy and reduced social functioning years later, yet retain the same diagnosis throughout. Attempts have been made to subdivide the syndrome into separate subgroups based on symptom clusters. The DSM and ICD classifications both include the subtypes of paranoid, disorganised, catatonic, undifferentiated and residual schizophrenia. Although these subtypes have a rich history, they do not seem to aggregate within families or predict prognosis (Kendler et al., 1994). More recently, attempts have been made to use statistical techniques such as factor analysis to generate subtypes, such as the 'deficit syndrome' (Kirkpatrick et al., 2001), but the level of agreement as to what constitutes these sub-syndromes is even less than for the overall syndrome of schizophrenia itself.

It is an interesting and useful exercise to consider what would happen if a completely naïve observer – the proverbial visitor from another planet – were to attempt a fresh classification of mental illnesses. Would he arrive at anything resembling the ICD or DSM? His classification would not necessarily be any better than ours, but I believe it would almost certainly be different. It is very likely that the classification would include at least one category of illness that shared many of the features of schizophrenia, since a large proportion of individuals receiving mental health care hear voices, harbour delusions and display deterioration in social functioning. However, it is possible to imagine many potential classifications that subdivided schizophrenia into many different but related disorders, and others that used a broader concept of schizophrenia (perhaps similar to the concept of 'psychosis' described below). Dimensional rather than categorical descriptions have been suggested, where individuals are seen as lying on a continuum between a complete absence of psychotic symptoms to severe illness.

How much does it matter how we define schizophrenia? My view is that many of the classifications proposed are more or less equally valid in scientific terms, so in some senses the question of how to classify schizophrenia could be viewed as a somewhat tedious and parochial debate among mental health professionals and researchers. However, there are two important areas where I believe that the definition of schizophrenia does matter.

The first is the problem of stigma. The label of schizophrenia is almost always seen in negative terms by patients and members of the public. To some extent this is inevitable, since, like cancer or stroke, schizophrenia is a devastating illness that has few, if any, positive aspects.

Some advocate changing the name of schizophrenia to something more palatable, although I am not convinced that this would have any more than a temporary impact on stigma, and it would inevitably create confusion. However, I would argue that because of the stigmatising nature of the illness, clinicians have a moral duty to ensure that the diagnosis is used as cautiously and precisely as possible.

The second problem is scientific validity. Unless researchers and clinicians can agree on an accepted definition, it is impossible to be sure that the results of a particular experiment or clinical trial are applicable to a particular patient, which is clearly vital if research is to have any clinical relevance.

In future, improved understanding of the genetics and aetiology of mental illnesses may allow us to devise a more valid classification. Until then, I believe the most pragmatic solution is to adhere as closely as possible to the clinical syndrome described in the classification systems. This at least has the advantage of maximising reliability (the extent to which different researchers are studying the same entity). This is essential if research is to add to an existing body of knowledge and be generalisable to clinical populations. However, it is important always to bear in mind that the concept of schizophrenia that we are employing is merely our current attempt to conceptualise a complex and confusing set of signs and symptoms, and to balance sometimes competing clinical, scientific and social priorities. Our concept of schizophrenia will probably evolve or be replaced as our knowledge and understanding of the disorder increases.

A note on terminology: psychosis

The word 'psychosis' is not defined in ICD–10, and it is used inconsistently in the literature and in clinical practice. In this book, I will use the word 'psychosis' to refer to the set of disorders listed in Table 4.11 on page 49, i.e. schizophrenia, schizoaffective disorder, bipolar affective disorder and other non-affective psychoses.

WHAT IS BIPOLAR DISORDER

Bipolar disorder is a mental disorder characterised primarily by acute episodes of grossly elevated and depressed mood, often with periods of relative stability in between episodes. Perceptual disturbances, delusions and thought disorder may occur. However, unlike schizophrenia, these disturbances tend to be congruent with the person's mood, and to recede when the mood returns to normal. Social, occupational and cognitive functioning are largely preserved, and emotions, far from being blunted as in schizophrenia, are usually exaggerated.

Definition

Several Greek physicians in the classical period recorded accounts of mania and melancholia, and Hippocrates wrote full descriptions of both conditions around 400 BC (Angst & Marneros, 2001). Aretaeus of Cappadocia was the first to link the two states as part of the same underlying disorder. In the mid-nineteenth century, the French concept of *folie circulaire*, coined by Jean-Pierre Falret at l'Hospice de la Sapêtrière, and Jules Baillarger's *folie à double forme* came very close to our modern conception of alternating states of mania and depression. However, these concepts were superseded for much of the twentieth century by Emil Kraepelin's notion in the 1890s of manic depressive insanity, which combined unipolar depression and bipolar mood disorders. The notion that bipolar disorder should be studied separately from unipolar depression was revived in the 1960s by Jules Angst and others, and the term *manic depressive psychosis* has been superseded by *bipolar disorder* in ICD–10 (WHO, 1992). However, unipolar and bipolar affective disorder were not clearly differentiated in ICD–9 (WHO, 1978), which combines 'major depressive disorder' with various categories of bipolar disorder under the heading 'affective psychosis'. For a discussion of how I have dealt with this issue in the SP_3 study, see page 64.

Hypomania

The term 'hypomania' refers to a mild state of mania. Although the definition of hypomania in ICD–10 allows for 'considerable interference with work or social activity', hypomania is often an asset. Hypomanic patients may work long and hard, be socially engaging and infectiously witty, and doggedly determined to achieve their goals. Some individuals profit greatly from this state, and hypomanic people are often very successful, particularly in business or creative occupations. However, at higher levels of mania, the person may become irritable, disorganised, indiscreet, promiscuous or aggressive, often with disastrous consequences such as marital break-up, redundancy, financial devastation or criminal proceedings. The difference between hypomania and mania is one of degree only, and the crucial distinction is the detrimental effect on social and occupational functioning that occurs with mania.

WHAT IS EPIDEMIOLOGY?

Epidemiology is the study of disorders at the population level, as opposed to the individual level. Epidemiology is primarily concerned with the incidence and prevalence of diseases in a population, and how these vary depending on risk factors. Population-based data can be very powerful (in both the technical sense of having the ability to demonstrate relatively small effects, and in colloquial sense of being persuasive and influencing policy makers). However, it is notoriously easy to draw erroneous conclusions from population-based data. Such data are often 'dirty': incomplete, collected by many different people, for purposes unrelated to the research, and in a sample that may not be representative of the population of interest. The discipline of epidemiology consists of the statistical and conceptual framework, with its associated caveats, for analysing and interpreting such data in as accurate and unbiased a manner as possible. In the words of the late epidemiologist Geoffrey Rose, epidemiologists should have dirty hands but clean minds.

THE EPIDEMIOLOGY OF SCHIZOPHRENIA

Age at onset

Schizophrenia often has an insidious onset, with deterioration in function occurring months or years before patients come to the attention of clinicians or researchers, so it can be difficult to define the moment of onset. The problem is compounded by the upper and lower age limits of many studies, which impose an artificial ceiling or floor on the range of possible ages. It is therefore difficult to obtain good estimates of the mean age of onset, but most studies place it in the late teens to mid-twenties, and schizophrenia is certainly rare before puberty. My colleague Helena Bundy and I have recently completed a meta-analysis (submitted for publication) showing that, regardless of the definition of onset, males develop schizophrenia between 1.8 and 2.6 years earlier than females (Bundy & MacCabe, in press). The reason for this gender difference is not understood.

Socioeconomic group

The findings on the association between socioeconomic indicators and schizophrenia are not completely clear. Although most studies have found associations between social deprivation at birth and schizophrenia (Castle et al., 1993; Harrison et al., 2001; Wicks et al., 2005), others have found associations with high socioeconomic status (Makikyro et al., 1997) or have found little relationship at all to socioeconomic group (Mulvany et al., 2001; Dutta, MacCabe et al., unpublished data).

Other (probably) social risk factors

A recent meta-analysis by McGrath and colleagues has shown that the incidence of schizophrenia varies up to fivefold in different settings (McGrath, 2006), contrary to the previously fashionable view that schizophrenia is a purely genetic disorder with a uniform distribution across the world.

Migrants have increased rates of schizophrenia, up to ninefold in some settings (Fearon et al., 2006), and this effect may be more pronounced for migrants from developing to developed countries. Furthermore, second generation migrants seem to be at least equally affected, and may even have higher rates than first generation migrants, suggesting that the increase in risk cannot be explained by risk factors surrounding migration itself, such as exposure to novel viruses or pollutants (Cantor-Graae & Selten, 2005). Although it remains possible that the causative agent may be purely biological (for example, prenatal vitamin D deficiency in dark-skinned migrants to temperate climates who are inadequately exposed to ultraviolet light during pregnancy (McGrath, 1999)) it is perhaps more likely to be related to psychological mechanisms associated with minority status (van Os et al., 2005). Supporting this proposition, Boydell and others have shown that black individuals in South London have the greatest risk if they live in predominantly white areas, suggesting that dissimilarity from the local community might be important (Boydell et al., 2001).

There is now abundant evidence that individuals from urban areas are at greater risk than those in rural areas, that this association cannot be explained by selective migration (Krabbendam & van Os, 2005), and that the critical period of exposure is probably during birth or early childhood, not at the time of illness onset (Marcelis et al., 1998). Again, the reasons for this association are obscure (McGrath & Scott, 2006), but social mechanisms seem more likely than biological ones.

The course and outcome of schizophrenia have also been found to vary between different populations. Of particular interest and concern to Western psychiatrists, there is some evidence that schizophrenia has a better social and functional outcome in developing countries, which often do not have access to pharmacological treatments (Hopper & Wanderling, 2000).

Early psychological trauma has recently come to attention as a risk factor for schizophrenia. Bebbington and colleagues (2004) found associations with a number of early victimisation experiences and adult schizophrenia, and studies by Agid et al. (1999) and Morgan et al. (2007) found associations with parental loss and separation. However, unlike most of the other epidemiological studies discussed here, these were all retrospective case–control studies, so the associations may be a result of recall bias.

Although infective agents, vitamin deficiencies and other biological causes have been postulated to explain these associations, all of these risk factors could reasonably be acting as proxies for chronic social adversity during childhood (van Os et al., 2005). It is not clear whether these social risk factors act via cognitive mechanisms, for example by establishing maladaptive attributional styles, or via biological processes, such as dysregulation of the hypothalamo–pituitary axis or the dopamine system.

Season of birth, prenatal and perinatal risk factors

There is consistent evidence for an excess of births of individuals who will develop schizophrenia in the winter and spring, although the effect seems weak or absent in the southern hemisphere (McGrath et al., 1995), and one very large population-based study failed to find an effect (Pedersen & Mortensen, 2001).

Pregnancy and birth complications appear to increase the risk of schizophrenia, and the range of insults appears to be very broad, including prematurity, perinatal hypoxia and Rhesus incompatibility (Cannon et al.,

2002a). In addition, several ecological studies have shown prenatal famine to be associated with schizophrenia in the offspring (St Clair et al., 2005).

Epidemiological studies have found that infection with influenza, rubella, toxoplasma gondii and herpes simplex virus type-2 during pregnancy are associated with increased risks for schizophrenia in the offspring (Brown, 2006). In one very impressive study using stored sera, Brown and colleagues (2004) found a risk ratio of seven for influenza in the first trimester.

Exposure to famine during pregnancy (in Holland in 1944–45, and in China in 1959–61) has also been associated with approximately double the risk of schizophrenia in the offspring.

Other studies have identified a range of maternal psychological stressors that appear to be prenatal risk factors for schizophrenia, including unwantedness of pregnancy (Myhrman et al., 1996) and exposure to military conflict (van Os & Selten, 1998) and natural disasters (Selten et al., 1999).

Cannabis and other drug use

There has been a recent explosion in research on the links between cannabis and schizophrenia. Although it has been very difficult to be certain of the direction of causality, the balance of evidence is now in favour of cannabis use as a risk factor for, rather than a consequence of, schizophrenia (van Os et al., 2005). Other drugs, including amphetamines (Curran et al., 2004), also appear to act as risk factors for schizophrenia.

Genetics of schizophrenia

Family, adoption and twin studies have shown that the risk of schizophrenia in the siblings and offspring of individuals with schizophrenia is around ten times the population rate. Heritability estimates for schizophrenia are consistently in the region of 80% (Owen et al., 2005), but the evidence suggests that, like many common disorders, schizophrenia is likely to have a complex mode of transmission, involving multiple genes.

Linkage and association studies (which aim to establish which particular genes are implicated in schizophrenia) have recently identified a growing number of candidate genes that are associated with increased risk for schizophrenia, particularly neuregulin (Li et al., 2006; Harrison & Law, 2006), dysbindin (Williams et al., 2005) and DISC-1 (Hodgkinson et al., 2004). However, these risk alleles individually produce only modest increases in risk for schizophrenia. It seems increasingly likely that there are many hundreds or even thousands of genetic variants that each have a relatively small effect on risk for schizophrenia at the population level.

Copy number variations

Recently, evidence has been accumulating that copy number variations (CNVs) may have an important role in the genetic architecture of schizophrenia. CNVs are stretches of DNA that are deleted or copied two or more times. A significant proportion of these may be mutations that have occurred very recently in evolutionary terms, and therefore affect only a small proportion of the population, or even just a single family. Recent mutations of this type are called *de novo* mutations.

The best studied CNV in schizophrenia is velo-cardio-facial syndrome (VCFS), also known as di George sequence or CATCH-22, a relatively common (population prevalence around 1:2000) deletion syndrome involving the deletion of 1.5–5.0 megabases in the 22q11.2 region. It follows an autosomal dominant pattern of inheritance, but the deletion occurs as a *de novo* mutation in around 90% of cases (Shprintzen, 2008). The clinical phenotype is very variable, but includes cardiac, palatal and facial anomalies, hypernasal speech, language delay, learning disabilities and psychiatric disorders (Robin & Shprintzen 2005). Psychosis occurs in around 30% of cases (Murphy et al., 1999). Of particular interest, the *catechol-O-methyltransferase* (*COMT*) gene is located in the deleted region. *COMT* is responsible for metabolising catecholamines, including dopamine, and has been studied extensively as a candidate gene for schizophrenia (Williams et al., 2007).

Four very recent studies, all using different designs, have provided evidence that schizophrenia is associated with *de novo* copy number variations more generally. Xu et al. (2008) studied 152 individuals with sporadic schizophrenia and 159 unaffected individuals. By comparing each individual with both parents, they performed a whole genome scan for gain or loss events, and found an eightfold increase in the frequency of new copy number variations in sporadic cases, compared with unaffected controls (15/152 compared with 2/159). Crucially, familial cases were not associated with *de novo* CNVs, suggesting that *de novo* CNV mutations may be a mechanism whereby new cases of schizophrenia enter the population.

Walsh and colleagues (2008) performed genome-wide scans in 418 individuals with schizophrenia and 268 healthy controls, for CNVs of >100 kilobases (kb). They identified 53 such CNVs that had not been previously reported, and these were three times more common in cases of schizophrenia than controls. Furthermore, the novel CNVs detected in the cases, but not those in controls, were overrepresented in pathways important in neurodevelopment (see section on neurodevelopmental theory, page 12).

Using a population-based sample of healthy parent–offspring pairs and trios (giving a total of 9878 transmissions), Stefansson et al. identified 66 *de novo* CNVs (Stefansson et al., 2008). They then tested these for association with schizophrenia in a sample of 1433 patients with psychosis and 33,250 controls, and found nominal associations in 3 CNVs, at 1q21.1, 15q11.2 and 15q13.3. Finally, they tested these three CNVs for association with psychosis in a further sample of 3285 cases and 7951 controls, and all three had significant associations.

In another study published simultaneously, the International Schizophrenia Consortium conducted a genome-wide search for CNVs in a sample of 3391 patients with schizophrenia and 3181 controls (2008). They identified 6753 CNVs of >100 kb that were present in less than 1%, and found that these were 1.15 times more common in patients than controls, and although subtle, this difference was highly significant ($p=3\times10^{-5}$). The authors identified three regions with excess large deletions in cases. These were at 22q11.2 (the VCFS region), and two of the regions identified in the Stefansson study above: namely, 1q21.1 and 22q11.2.

These data imply that rare *de novo* mutations are responsible for a higher proportion of the genetic risk for schizophrenia than previously assumed, perhaps specifically sporadic cases. Some regions, such as 22q11.2, 1q21.1 and 15q13.3, seem to be particularly associated with large deletions. However, it also appears that rare *de novo* CNVs in a wide variety of regions, are also capable of causing schizophrenia, particularly in regions containing genes relating to neurodevelopment. If this is the case, then rare, *de novo* CNVs may explain the familial transmission of schizophrenia within some families, and high concordance rates between monozygotic (MZ) twins, yet have little or no association with schizophrenia at the population level. This may help to explain the disappointing progress in identifying risk variants for schizophrenia despite high heritability. It may also explain the fact that schizophrenia persists in the population despite clear selection pressure against it (MacCabe et al., 2009): thus it could be that there is a strong selection pressure acting against CNVs that predispose to schizophrenia, but this negative selection is balanced by a constant supply of new CNVs into the gene pool.

Genes, environments and interactions

Many of the environmental risk factors associated with schizophrenia, such as migration, urban birth and prenatal viral infections, seem to be more strongly associated with schizophrenia than any known genetic variant, even though most of these environmental factors are probably only proxy measures. This presents two conundrums. First, given the ubiquity of many of these environmental risk factors, such as urban birth and cannabis use, how do the majority of the exposed population manage to evade schizophrenia? Second, how can these large risk ratios for environmental factors be reconciled with the evidence that schizophrenia has over 80% heritability (Cardno et al., 1999)?

One explanation with great explanatory power, and with a small but growing body of evidence, is that vulnerability to environmental agents may be heritable – so-called genotype–environment interaction. Probably the best evidence for genotype–environmental interaction in schizophrenia is in relation to cannabis use. Caspi and colleagues (2005) recently showed that homozygotes for the Val allele of the *catechol-O-methyltransferase* (*COMT*) Val(158)Met polymorphism were at increased risk for psychosis if they took cannabis, whereas cannabis did not appear to influence risk in Met–Met homozygotes. Cannabis had an intermediate effect in heterozygotes. In an experimental study, Henquet and others showed that carriers of the Val allele were more likely to experience psychotic experiences and impairments in memory and attention when exposed to Delta-9-tetrahydrocannabidiol, the principal psychotropic compound in cannabis smoke (Henquet et al., 2006a).

As well as genotype–environment interactions, it is possible there are gene–gene interactions (whereby a gene variant only increases risk for schizophrenia in the presence of another variant), genotype–environmental correlations (genotype influences the probability of exposure to an environmental agent), and environment–environment interactions. The psychiatric epidemiologist Ezra Susser has argued that risks resulting from gene–environment interactions and correlations tend to be attributed to genes in most genetic epidemiological studies, so that if such effects are operating, it is likely that heritability estimates will be exaggerated (Schwartz & Susser, 2006).

The neurodevelopmental theory of schizophrenia

Until the mid-1980s, schizophrenia was thought to involve a neurodegenerative process. However, neuropathological, epidemiological, cognitive and neuroimaging evidence began to suggest that schizophrenia may instead be associated with a relatively static neuropathology, arising early in life, that predisposed the individual to express the disorder in adulthood. Schizophrenia was thus reformulated as a neurodevelopmental disorder (Murray & Lewis, 1987; Weinberger, 1987) and this model has now gained wide acceptance. In its current form, the neurodevelopmental theory of schizophrenia proposes that genetic, and/or early environmental factors disrupt brain development *in utero*, resulting in impaired neurodevelopment throughout childhood, and that this neurodevelopmental impairment results in subtle social and cognitive problems, and puts the individual at enhanced risk of psychosis from adolescence onwards. The mechanism by which neurodevelopmental impairment might predispose to psychosis is not understood in detail. One possibility is that neurodevelopmental impairment may sensitise individuals to the effects of environmental risk factors in childhood and adolescence, such as psychosocial stress and drug misuse (Dean et al., 2003).

THE EPIDEMIOLOGY OF BIPOLAR DISORDER

Age at onset and sex distribution

Age at onset is even more difficult to study in bipolar disorder than in schizophrenia, since the diagnosis is not made until at least one episode of mania has occurred, which may be long after the first depressive episode. A recent epidemiological study of mania in London found that incidence peaked between the ages of 21 and 25, with 17% occurring before age 20 (Kennedy et al., 2005a). Males had an earlier onset by about 5 years. Most studies have found little or no sex difference in incidence or prevalence, or a slight excess of females (Kennedy et al., 2005b).

Socioeconomic group

As with schizophrenia, there has been little research into the association between socioeconomic group and bipolar disorder, but in the case of bipolar disorder, the findings are more consistent. Early studies found that bipolar patients, despite being socially disadvantaged themselves, came from families of high socioeconomic status (Hirschfeld & Cross, 1982). This has been confirmed in more recent case–control studies (Verdoux & Bourgeois, 1995; Abood et al., 2002), and in large population-based studies (Aro et al., 1995; Tsuchiya et al., 2004).

Other (probably) social risk factors

Compared with schizophrenia, there have been few studies on the environmental risk factors for bipolar disorder. In general, most of the studies that have investigated whether known risk factors for schizophrenia are also risk factors for bipolar disorder have been negative.

Marcelis and colleagues (1998) found a very modest (incidence rate ratio (IRR) 1.18, 95% CI 1.15 to 1.21) association between urban birth and bipolar disorder in the Netherlands, but two studies from Denmark (Mortensen et al., 2003; Pedersen & Mortensen, 2006), found no such association.

With regard to ethnicity and migration, a recent meta-analysis estimated the risk ratio for bipolar disorder to be around 2.5 in migrants (Swinnen & Selten, 2007). However, much of this excess was attributable to African–Caribbean people in the UK, who have been found to have extremely high rates of both schizophrenia and mania (Kirkbride et al., 2006). Indeed, when the contribution of African–Caribbean people in the UK was removed from the meta-analysis described above, the risk was no longer significantly increased (Swinnen & Selten, 2007).

In a national Danish sample, Mortensen and colleagues (2003) found that children who lost their mother early had an excess of bipolar disorder in adulthood, approximately fourfold for maternal loss in the first 5 years. An earlier case–control study by Agid and colleagues (1999) had produced similar findings.

Recent life events and stress have been linked to the onset of bipolar disorder in several retrospective studies, although it has not yet been possible to assess this association in prospective studies (Johnson, 2005).

Season of birth, prenatal and perinatal risk factors

In a large case–control study, Torrey and colleagues found an excess of winter births for bipolar disorder, which was greater than that for depression (Torrey et al., 1996). Hultman and colleagues found a similar association in a Swedish register-based study (Hultman et al., 1999), although Mortensen's large Danish population study did not replicate this finding (Pedersen & Mortensen, 2001). The Danish study also found no association with influenza *in utero*, but, to my knowledge, no other prenatal infections have been studied as risk factors for bipolar disorder. Both Hultman and Mortensen conducted large cohort studies examining measures of foetal growth and hypoxia as risk indicators for bipolar disorder, and neither found an association (Hultman et al., 1999; Ogendahl et al., 2006), although Hultman found a modest effect for uterine atony.

Cannabis and other drug use

Bipolar disorder is associated with the use of a range of psychoactive drugs including cannabis (Strakowski et al., 2007), but the large cohort studies in Sweden and New Zealand that have demonstrated the associations between adolescent cannabis use and schizophrenia have tended to focus on schizophrenia or psychotic symptoms, but not on bipolar disorder. However, one recent prospective study showed a modest excess of bipolar disorder after 3 years in people who reported cannabis use (Henquet et al., 2006b).

Genetics of bipolar disorder

Heritability estimates of bipolar disorder are typically very similar to those of schizophrenia, at just over 80% (Cardno et al., 1999). Recently, the first putative genetic variants have been associated with bipolar, and these are discussed on pages 16–17.

SCHIZOPHRENIA AND BIPOLAR DISORDER: DIVISION VERSUS OVERLAP

The Kraepelinian divide

It is doubtful whether even Emil Kraepelin himself could have foreseen the impact of his distinction between 'dementia praecox' and 'manic depressive insanity' on the history of psychiatry.

Kraepelin's key contribution was the realisation that the course and prognosis of patients with psychotic disorders was associated with the pattern of symptoms. In particular, prominent mood symptoms seemed to confer a good prognosis. The attempt to classify mental illnesses was undoubtedly an important step forward for the scientific study of psychiatry. It also performed useful functions in clinical practice, by allowing more accurate prognosis, and probably also by facilitating the development of treatments for mood disorders and psychotic symptoms.

Kraepelin was careful to emphasise that what distinguished the disorders was not any particular pathognomonic symptom, but rather a pattern of symptoms; thus there is hardly any symptom that may appear in one disorder but not in the other. However, the division between schizophrenia and bipolar disorder became more marked over time, and a century later, almost all psychiatric textbooks, and both major classification systems, have separate chapters for 'psychoses' and 'affective disorders'.

It is easy to imagine how attractive Kraepelin's classification must have been from scientific, political and clinical perspectives. In the fledgling discipline of psychiatry, classification was rightly seen as a necessary step on the road to scientific acceptability, and Kraepelin's method itself, consisting of the synthesis of information from many years of meticulous clinical observations, could be seen as a kind of scientific process. Politically, psychiatry was struggling to gain acceptance as a medical specialty, and the ability to make diagnoses was important in establishing credibility in mainstream medicine. Clinically, the idea that the confusing morass of insanity could be neatly divided into two categories was presumably appealing, and the ability to make predictions about the course of illness from a patient's presenting symptoms was undoubtedly an important development.

However, Kraepelin's system seems to ignore the inconvenient fact that psychiatrists frequently encounter patients with a mixture of affective and schizophrenic symptoms, who do not fall neatly into either category. The psychiatric profession, in my opinion, has been astonishingly inventive in finding ways to maintain the Kraepelinian dichotomy in the face of evidence against it.

The crudest approach was to adopt a hierarchical approach to diagnosis, whereby schizophrenia 'trumps' mood disorders, so patients exhibiting symptoms of both disorders are simply classified as suffering from schizophrenia, with the mood disorder assumed to be a secondary effect.

The introduction of a separate diagnostic category of schizoaffective disorder was at least an acknowledgement that intermediate patients exist. But this may even have reinforced the existence of archetypal schizophrenic and bipolar groups in the minds of psychiatrists, by protecting both these classical groups from 'contamination' by patients who exhibited mixed symptoms. In any case, schizoaffective disorder has been very infrequently used in some settings, particularly in Scandinavian countries, where schizoaffective disorder is viewed by many psychiatrists as a temporary category, to be used only until the true diagnosis becomes clear. Many psychiatrists have been trained to believe that schizoaffective disorder is the refuge of the poor diagnostician, who, lacking the skill or confidence to commit to a 'definite' diagnosis, sits on the fence. In research, schizoaffective disorder has hardly ever been taken seriously as a diagnostic category, and patients who do not conform to the standard notions of schizophrenia or bipolar disorder are either not included in research studies, or shoe-horned into one or other category.

Unitary psychosis model

For many years there has been an undercurrent of dissent from the prevailing dichotomous view (Kendell & Gourlay, 1970; Brockington et al., 1979; Crow, 1990). Initially, the emphasis was on the phenomenology (pattern of symptoms) of the two disorders, such as the studies of Kendell and colleagues (Kendell & Gourlay, 1970; Brockington et al., 1979), which used statistical techniques to try to validate the Kraepelinian dichotomy, but instead found evidence for a continuum (the so-called 'unitary psychosis' model), with many patients displaying a mixture of symptoms.

Evidence from twin and family studies has also shown that bipolar disorder occurs at higher rates in the relatives of individuals with schizophrenia, and vice versa (Craddock et al., 2006; Mortensen et al., 2003), and studies that have studied schizoaffective disorder have found that it is genetically related to both disorders (Kendler et al., 1998).

Genetic studies may have underestimated the overlap between the schizophrenia and bipolar disorder by using the hierarchical diagnostic system. Alistair Cardno and colleagues showed that, when the diagnostic hierarchy for psychiatric disorders is suspended, there is a strong overlap in genetic risk for schizophrenia and bipolar disorder (Cardno et al., 2002).

This overlap is now supported by molecular genetic studies, which have implicated three genetic variants that are also associated with schizophrenia: namely, *DAOA* (formerly called *G72/G30*), *DISC-1*, *NRG-1*, and found suggestive evidence in several others, including *COMT* and *BDNF* (Farmer et al., 2007).

Bipolar disorder and schizophrenia also have neuropharmacological similarities. Antipsychotic drugs, which act predominantly to reduce meso-limbic dopamine transmission, have recently been shown to be effective in bipolar disorder as well as schizophrenia (Tohen et al., 2006).

Important differences

There is no denying that classical cases of schizophrenia and bipolar disorder do exist, and patients at either end of the schizophrenia/bipolar spectrum do differ from one another in important ways. As I have outlined above, schizophrenia seems to be associated with a range of perinatal abnormalities that do not seem to act as risk factors for bipolar disorder. Differences in brain structure also exist, particularly reductions in total brain volume, grey matter volume and in the volumes of medial temporal lobe structures, all of which are found in schizophrenia but not in bipolar disorder. In the amygdala, there is evidence of increased volume in bipolar disorder, but reduced volume in schizophrenia (Murray et al., 2004).

Probably the most consistent difference is that patients with predomin-antly bipolar symptoms have better cognitive functioning than those with schizophrenia, both before and after illness onset. In addition, children who will develop schizophrenia have abnormal social and motor development prior to the onset of schizophrenia, but this is not the case for those who develop bipolar disorder. I will review the data on premorbid function in schizophrenia and bipolar disorder in detail in Chapter 3.

The neurodevelopmental theory to the rescue?

So far I have argued that schizophrenia and bipolar disorder are best seen as the extremes of a spectrum of psychosis, but that the distinctions between classical bipolar and schizophrenia are real and important. Any aetiological model that successfully explains psychosis will have to take the overlap and distinctions between schizophrenia and bipolar disorder into account.

It seems likely that that certain risk factors predispose an individual to psychosis generally; for example, genes like *DISC-1*, *DAOA* and *NRG-1* and some environmental risk factors, such as minority status and cannabis consumption, may fall into this category. Other genes and environmental risk factors probably determine the extent to which schizophrenic or bipolar symptoms predominate. For example, pregnancy and birth com-plications seem to be specific to schizophrenia, and children who go on to develop schizophrenia have a wide range of developmental delays and cognitive deficits that are either absent or much milder in bipolar disorder.

Risk factors specific to bipolar disorder are fewer, but higher socioeconomic group seems to be a consistent risk factor.

But can the difference between the risk factors for bipolar and schizophrenia give us any clues about aetiology? It is notable that most of the differences involve abnormalities that are present in schizophrenia but not bipolar disorder. This may be because bipolar is much less heavily researched than schizophrenia. However, it suggests that schizophrenia might be the result of an additional insult that is not present in bipolar disorder.

One possibility is that the difference between the two disorders is related to disrupted neurodevelopment (Demjaha et al., in press). This is consistent with the fact that schizophrenia, but not bipolar disorder, seems to be associated with pre-morbid cognitive, social and motor deficits, and with brain structural abnormalities such as reduced whole brain, grey matter and medial temporal lobe volumes. The fact that some schizophrenia risk factors, such as hypoxia and prenatal viral infections, have a biologically plausible link with neurodevelopment, adds weight to this argument.

CHAPTER TWO

Intelligence, creativity and mental illness

Great wits are sure to madness near allied,
And thin partitions do their bounds divide.
(John Dryden, 1681/2004)

So observed John Dryden in 1681 in *Absalom and Achitophel*. The belief in an association between madness and creativity can be found in the writings of Aristotle, Plato and Socrates (Hershman and Lieb, 1998).

This notion is very seductive. For those with mental illness, the possibility that their suffering may be associated with superior abilities is a source of optimism. For artists, the model of the anguished genius, as personified by Lord Byron, Vincent van Gogh and others, has served as a romantic ideal for centuries. In popular culture, archetypes such as the tormented artist, the mad scientist, even the depressive comic genius, are widespread. One possible explanation for the endurance of this notion is that people are particularly receptive to ideas that seem counter-intuitive, selectively remembering information that is surprising or paradoxical (Boyer & Ramble, 2001).

Whatever the reason for its appeal, what is the evidence for the association? Examples abound of creative individuals who have suffered from mental illness, from Vincent van Gogh (Jamison, 1993) to John Nash (Nasar, 1998), but these tell us merely that it is possible to have mental illness and also be creative, not that the two are related (David, 1999).

METHODOLOGICAL DIFFICULTIES

There are several difficulties inherent in studying links between creativity and psychiatric illness.

Defining creativity

When writing about measuring creativity, the psychologist Hans Eysenck described how he found himself being 'allusive' and 'overinclusive' because 'creativity is a very complex subject' (Eysenck, 1994). The following definition contains the two important elements found in most definitions of creativity: 'Creativity denotes a person's capacity to produce new or original ideas, insights, inventions, or artistic products, which are accepted by experts as being of scientific, aesthetic, social or technical value' (Vernon, 1989). One component in most definitions of creativity is novelty, or 'improbable combinations of old ideas' (Eysenck, 1994). Another is that creative ideas must also be valuable (Eysenck, 1994).

Subjectivity

Deciding whether an idea or a piece of art has sufficient novelty and value to be considered creative is clearly a highly subjective task. Much of the research in this area has also used subjective techniques to abstract evidence of mental illness and failed to distinguish between different types of psychopathology. Only a few recent studies have used operationalised definitions of schizophrenia or bipolar disorder.

Rarity

By definition, exceptional creativity must be rare. The mental disorders of interest here, particularly schizophrenia and bipolar disorder, are also rare. The ideal study to assess the presence and strength of any association between mental disorder and creativity would take a representative sample of the population, measure both creativity and mental disorder, and then examine the relationship between these two rare factors at the population level. However, the rarity of both creativity and mental disorder means that such a study would require very large samples. Much of the literature, therefore, uses small, case–control designs, with their inherent methodological weaknesses.

Bias

Bias is any deviation of the results or inferences of a study from the truth, which leads to conclusions that are systematically different from the truth (Last, 2001).

Most of the case–control studies described above are biographical studies. In these studies, the lives of eminent individuals are scrutinised, often posthumously, for evidence of mental illness. Thus, in addition to the general problems outlined above, biographical studies suffer from the following biases.

Selection bias

Selection bias refers to a situation in which the selection of participants in the study occurs in such a way that the result is biased. For example, in many studies investigating associations between creativity and psychosis, the individuals to be studied are hand-picked by the author, with the obvious risk that, whether consciously or unconsciously, the author will favour individuals whose histories will confirm their hypotheses. In some studies, attempts are made to reduce selection bias through the use of independent (although ultimately still subjective) criteria for inclusion such as awards and other accolades of esteem rather than the judgement of the researcher; others have used more subjective criteria such as enhanced skills and ability to achieve increased social status as markers of creativity.

Information bias

Information bias in this context is a bias in the selection or abstraction of information from biographical material. This can occur at several levels. The biographer himself may favour facts that emphasise the dramatic connections between mental distress and creativity, and his sources may themselves be biased in this way. The researcher may also introduce bias, in deciding which material to include or emphasise.

TYPES OF STUDY DESIGN

Four broad types of study design have attempted to address the question empirically: historical or biographical studies, case–control studies of mental illness in living individuals who are identified as gifted, case–control studies measuring creativity or similar characteristics in clinical samples and population-based studies. In addition, some of the above designs have been extended to the relatives of index cases.

Biographical studies and case series

Although intrinsically fascinating, these studies are fraught with problems, as discussed above: they are subjective, retrospective studies on biased samples with no comparison group and usually no first-hand information about the individual, let alone clinical information.

An example was the study of Jamison (1989), which described the biographies of 47 writers and artists and found that 38% had received treatment for mood disorders at some time in their lives. Indeed, almost all these studies found greater than expected rates of mental illness in gifted or creative people, but had severe methodological flaws (Waddell, 1998).

One biographical study that attempted to use control groups was that of Ludwig (1992), who reviewed biographies of over a thousand individuals from creative and non-creative occupations. Those in vocations that were judged to be creative had over twice the rates of depression compared with those in business, science or public life.

Studies of mental illness in gifted individuals

Nancy Andreasen and colleagues were the first to undertake a modern study using detailed psychiatric assessments and standardised diagnostic criteria, in living creative individuals. The authors compared a group of 30 writers on the prestigious Iowa Writers' Workshop with a group of age, education and sex-matched controls. They found very much higher rates of affective disorder generally, particularly bipolar disorder (43% versus 10%) and alcoholism among the writers compared with the controls. There were no cases of schizophrenia in either group. In addition, they found elevated rates of mood disorders in the siblings of the writers, compared with those of controls (Andreasen, 1987).

Another study by Ludwig (1994) compared 59 female writers with 59 members of a matched comparison group, using interviews and questionnaires. The writers were more likely than the comparison group to suffer from mood disorders, and similar effects were seen for substance misuse and anxiety disorders.

Studies of giftedness in individuals with mental illness

Richards and colleagues measured lifetime creativity in patients with bipolar disorder, cyclothymia (a milder category of bipolar mood disorder, commonly diagnosed in the USA) and 'controls', who comprised a mixture of patients with other psychiatric disorders and well individuals. They failed to show any statistical differences between the groups (Richards et al., 1988).

Population-based studies

Icelandic studies

In a research programme lasting over 30 years, Jon Karlsson has used Icelandic case registers to study associations between mental illness and a number of measures of high functioning (Karlsson, 2004). In one study, he compared individuals with exceptionally good academic functioning (the top two individuals in the country each year) at approximately 18 years of age to the remainder of the population. He showed that these individuals were at increased risk of psychosis, and their first-degree relatives, particularly their siblings, were also at high risk. In a later analysis, it appeared that high achievers in mathematics and their relatives were at particularly high risk.

There are several problems with these studies. First, psychosis is treated as a unitary category and is not precisely defined. Second, despite the large number of individuals studied, the numbers were very small in each of these comparisons. The number of cases of psychosis expected in the 180 top graduates was 1.4, and the observed number was 4. Although this suggests an association, it is hardly persuasive evidence.

The 1966 Northern Finland Birth Cohort study

This cohort of 11,000 individuals, with prospectively collected information on school performance, was followed using the Finnish Hospital Discharge Register until 1994, when the cohort were 28 years old. The outcomes of interest were schizophrenia, other psychoses and non-psychotic psychiatric disorders.

The authors used two measures of poor school functioning: a categorical variable indicating that the student was not in his expected class at age 14, and the grade-point average achieved at age 16 among those who were in their normal class.

Boys with excellent school performance at age 16 had a fourfold increased risk of schizophrenia compared with controls. However, again the numbers were small, and if two fewer cases of schizophrenia had occurred in the excellent performance group, the result would not have been statistically significant. Furthermore, the effect was completely absent in girls (Isohanni et al., 1999).

Israeli studies

Like the Scandinavian countries, Israel has a well-developed system of registers that can be linked using national identification numbers. In 1999, Michael Davidson and colleagues published a nested case–control study, in which 509 patients with schizophrenia were matched on age, gender and school to 9215 controls; each case was matched to the mean score of the remainder of his class, and the analysis was a matched design using conditional logistic regression (Davidson et al., 1999). Only boys were included. Conscription occurred at age 16–17 between 1985 and 1991 and follow-up continued until 1995, when the cohort were aged approximately 20–27.

The proportion of pre-schizophrenia cases falling within the highest IQ category among the cases was six times higher than that among the comparison subjects (Davidson et al., 1999).

Dunedin cohort

In the Dunedin Multidisciplinary Health and Development Study, a 1-year birth cohort from 1972–73 was assessed at biennial intervals between ages 3 and 11 on a range of emotional, behavioural and interpersonal problems, motor and language development, and intelligence (Cannon et al., 2002b). Study participants were asked about psychotic symptoms at age 11 and were interviewed at age 26, using a diagnostic interview schedule. Only a small proportion met criteria for schizophrenia, partly because of the requirement, under DSM–IV, for 6 months chronicity. The broader category of schizophreniform disorder was therefore used instead, yielding 36 cases. In addition, mania was used as an outcome (n=20).

Children who would develop mania in adulthood performed significantly better than controls on motor performance, even after controlling for sex and socioeconomic status. Very recently, the same researchers showed that these children who will go on to develop mania also had significantly higher IQs than the remainder of the cohort, but the authors acknowledged that the sample was small, with only 8 children who would go on to develop mania, and they called for replications in a larger sample (Koenen et al., 2009).

Studies of the relatives of patients with psychosis

Patients with schizophrenia have greatly impaired fertility (MacCabe et al., 2009), raising the question of how this strongly genetic disorder does not simply die out over a few generations. It has been proposed that creative cognitive styles may share a genetic basis with severe mental disorders, and that creativity may enhance reproductive fitness in patients' relatives (Nettle, 2001). Some studies in the 1990s suggested the relatives of people diagnosed with schizophrenia might indeed have slightly enhanced fertility (Fananas & Bertranpetit 1995; Srinivasan & Padmavati 1997). However, more recently, our research group compared the number of offspring in a birth cohort of over 12,000 Swedish people, who were born between 1915 and 1929, and followed up for over two generations (MacCabe et al., 2009). We showed that, while patients with schizophrenia had very low fertility, the unaffected siblings and children of the people with schizophrenia (n=58), or affective psychosis (n=153) had no more offspring than the remainder of the population. A meta-analysis by my colleague Helena Bundy, combining data from all population-based studies comparing fertility in the unaffected siblings of people with schizophrenia with that of the general population, has since confirmed that the relatives of people with schizophrenia have entirely normal fertility (Bundy & MacCabe, 2009, in press). These data make the hypothesis that schizophrenia persists through enhanced creativity leading to increased fertility in the relatives completely untenable. Nevertheless, the hypothesis has led to a number of studies on creativity in the relatives of patients with psychosis.

Karlsson's more recent studies in Iceland are described on page 22. In an earlier study, he examined the achievements of the first-degree relatives of people with a history of psychosis. He found an excess of authors, holders of doctorates, professors, parliamentarians and clergyman among these relatives. They were also around 30% more likely than the general population to be listed in the Icelandic version of *Who's Who* (Karlsson, 1984).

Tom McNeil (1971) examined the psychiatric diagnostic status of creative Danish adoptees, their first-degree biological relatives and their adopted relatives. Three judges rated the adoptees as creative or non-creative on the basis of their occupation, and went on to rate individuals as to the degree of their creativity. The researchers identified the adoptees, and their biological and adoptive parents in a register of people who had been treated for psychiatric disorders.

From over 5000 potential adoptees, 50 were included and 10 of these were described as 'highly creative'. Five of the 10 adoptees judged highly creative had been treated for mental disorder, compared with 0 out of the 20 judged to demonstrate low creativity. When the researchers examined the rates of mental disorders in the adoptive and biological parents, they found that overall, the biological parents of the adoptees were more likely to have been treated for psychiatric disorders than the adoptive parents. This is hardly surprising, since the adoptive parents were presumably screened for mental health problems prior to adopting, and in some cases, mental disorder in the biological parents would have been the reason for adoption. However, the probability of mental health problems in the biological parents was strongly associated with the creativity of the offspring, whereas the probability of mental disorder in the adoptive parents was unrelated to creativity in the adoptees. These results suggested that there was a genetic association between creativity and mental disorder, although the methodology and statistical analysis would be judged as flawed by today's standards.

Kinney and colleagues conducted a similar study using Danish adoptees, but on this occasion they looked for evidence of enhanced creativity amongst 36 adoptees who had already been established to have a high genetic loading for schizophrenia-spectrum disorders (Kinney et al., 2001). The researchers blindly assessed transcripts of the interviews with these adoptees, using a standardised creativity scale. Fifteen of the adopted offspring of parents with schizophrenia showed evidence of schizoid personality disorder or schizotypal disorder. These 15 also had higher scores for creativity when compared with asymptomatic control adoptees (2.03 (SD=0.69) versus 1.83 (SD=0.65) p=ns).

CONCLUSION

So what can we conclude from the studies described in this chapter? We can be certain from case reports that it is possible to have either schizophrenia or bipolar disorder and also be exceptionally talented in a particular domain. The weight of evidence from the biographical and case–control studies suggests that there is probably an association between mood disorder, and being in a creative occupation. The evidence seems strongest for an association between bipolar disorder and creative writing. However, the direction of cause and effect cannot be determined.

The population-based studies all use different measures of academic achievement or cognitive performance, and are mostly confined to men. However, these population studies, although far from conclusive, also suggest the presence of an association, for schizophrenia, bipolar disorder or psychosis generally.

CHAPTER THREE

Pre-morbid neuropsychological functioning in schizophrenia and bipolar disorder: a review of the published literature

There have been hundreds of studies examining neuropsychological functioning in schizophrenia and bipolar disorder. However, the vast majority of these have used cross-sectional, case–control designs to compare people with schizophrenia or bipolar disorder with unaffected controls on measures of current cognitive functioning. Heinrichs and Zakzanis (1998) summarised the results of over 200 studies on cognitive function in schizophrenia and concluded that schizophrenia was characterised by a broadly based cognitive impairment, which affected all domains tested to varying degrees. In the case of bipolar disorder, deficits tend to be much milder (Krabbendam et al., 2005), but patients do exhibit deficits in executive function and verbal memory, even between illness episodes (Robinson et al., 2006).

The main difficulty with interpreting these studies is that any deficits found could have arisen through any combination of at least five possible mechanisms.

1. They could have been involved in the aetiology (causation) of the disorder, in which case one would expect them to predate the onset of illness.
2. They could be a core symptom of the disorder itself, and/or the result of a neurodegenerative process.
3. They could be secondary to the symptoms of psychosis (distraction by auditory hallucinations, mood changes, agitation, apathy etc.).
4. They could be secondary to the treatment for psychosis.

5. They could be secondary to the chronically impoverished social and
    occupational environment of many patients with chronic mental illness.

The difficulty with retrospective and cross-sectional studies is that it is very
difficult to establish how long any cognitive deficits have been present. One
cannot distinguish pre-morbid deficits (i.e. deficits that pre-date the onset of
illness) from deficits arising from the other four causes.

Other well-recognised problems with retrospective and cross-sectional
research designs include selection bias (the selection of a non-representative
sample of cases and/or controls) and recall bias (the tendency for cases and
controls to report their previous history differently).

Most of these problems can be overcome by using a prospective research
design. In a prospective design, cognitive function is measured in childhood or adolescence, prior to the onset of psychosis, and the subjects are
followed-up over time to establish which of them developed psychosis.

Since I am interested in the aetiology of psychosis, I will therefore
restrict my review to high-quality studies that have used prospective designs
to measure intellectual functioning before the onset of disorder. As it
happens, all of these studies have used historical cohort designs or nested
case–control designs within historical cohorts (these study designs are
explained in detail starting on page 41). This means that the data were
collected prospectively, on a well-defined cohort of people, so that from the
point of view of eliminating bias, the data for the 'exposure' (cognitive
functioning) are uncontaminated by knowledge of the outcome (psychosis).
In a traditional cohort study, the researchers would have been involved in
the collection of the data for exposure, and in monitoring the cohort over
time to measure the outcome. However, in a historical cohort study, the
data are collected in the absence of the researcher, usually for a completely
different purpose, and the researchers collate and analyse the data after
both the exposure and the outcome have occurred.

Rather than recount an exhaustive list of papers, I have selected the
largest and most relevant studies in the field, and although this is a selective
review, I am confident that I have not omitted any major studies that fulfil
these criteria. Where the results from a cohort have been reported in more
than one paper, I have grouped the results together.

MASON, 1956

Probably the first study to address this question prospectively was that of
Mason in 1956. Mason used scores from routine US Army tests during
World War II (it is not clear exactly what these measured) and clinical
diagnoses from a single hospital. He compared scores from the various
diagnostic groups with those from a control group comprising almost

300,000 men from the same geographical area. Patients with schizophrenia achieved significantly lower scores than the control group, while manic–depressive patients scored significantly higher than expected. Although Mason's methodology was very advanced for its time, it is difficult to draw inferences from this study as the clinical concept of schizophrenia was much broader in the USA in the 1950s than it is today.

THE BRITISH BIRTH COHORT STUDIES

National Survey of Health and Development (1946 birth cohort)

In 1994, Peter Jones and colleagues published a study on a birth cohort of 5362 people born in a single week in 1946 and given a broad range of cognitive tests at ages 8, 11 and 15 years (Jones et al., 1994). They were then followed up between age 16 and 43 by regular contacts with the research team. In addition, a national register of admissions to psychiatric hospitals in Britain from 1974 to 1986 (the Mental Health Enquiry) was used to identify additional cases. There were 30 cases of schizophrenia overall. Children who were to subsequently develop schizophrenia scored consistently lower on all measures of cognitive function, particularly on non-verbal tests, and there appeared to be an approximately linear association between cognitive score and risk for schizophrenia. This association did not appear to be confounded by socioeconomic group or sex (see page 97 for a definition of confounding). There was a tendency for the disparity between individuals who would later develop schizophrenia and healthy individuals to increase with age.

Jim van Os and colleagues performed a similar analysis on the same cohort (1997), and found that children who would later have affective disorders also underperformed on these tests, but to a lesser extent. The study did not differentiate between future cases of unipolar and bipolar disorder, but it seems that unipolar cases predominated (Murray, RM, personal communication).

National Child Development Survey (1958 birth cohort)

This survey followed a very similar design to the 1946 birth cohort discussed above, although it relied exclusively on the Mental Health Enquiry for retrieval of cases (Done et al., 1994). The subjects were only 28 years old at the end of follow-up, so the study was probably biased in favour of early-onset cases. The 40 children who would go on to develop schizophrenia in adulthood showed a stable pattern of deficits at 7 and 11 years of around 0.6–0.7 standard deviations across a wide range of neuropsychological assessments and subjective teachers' ratings of school work. Again, children who would later develop affective psychosis had a smaller deficit, but there was no distinction between unipolar and bipolar disorder (Jones and Done, 1997).

SWEDISH CONSCRIPT STUDIES

David et al., 1997

In 1997, Anthony David and colleagues studied data from 50,000 males conscripted into the Swedish army from 1969 to 1970 at age 18, who underwent cognitive tests at conscription (David et al., 1997). This was the first study of this type to make use of the Scandinavian registers of routinely collected data, which can be linked by means of the personal identification numbers carried by all citizens. The study linked data from the Swedish Army to the Swedish National Register of Psychiatric Care, which contained data on all admitted cases of schizophrenia in Sweden until 1984. In total 195 cases of schizophrenia, and 192 of other psychoses (including bipolar disorder but also unipolar depression and other non-affective psychoses), were identified. Low overall IQ was highly predictive of both outcomes, particularly for schizophrenia.

These associations persisted after controlling for socioeconomic status, behavioural adjustment in childhood, drug misuse, urban upbringing, family history of psychiatric disorder and psychiatric disturbance at the time of testing. Mechanical knowledge showed the strongest association with schizophrenia, and was the only one of four domains that remained significantly associated with schizophrenia after adjustment for the other three domains.

The authors also compared the distributions of scores in patients and the population, and there was no evidence of a low-performing subgroup. There was, however, some evidence that the risk in the lowest category was greater than would have been expected in a statistically linear association, although a likelihood ratio test for departure from linear trend was only significant in the 'other psychoses' group.

Although it is important to assess whether a low-performing subgroup is responsible for the association, it is difficult to interpret statistical tests of departure from linear trend, since these cognitive test scores are not strictly continuous variables. In other words, the difference between scoring, say, 3 and 4 on one of the Swedish Army's tests of cognitive ability does not necessarily represent the same disparity in cognitive performance as the difference between, say, 7 and 8, even though both represent an increase of one on the scale.

Zammit et al., 2004

In 2004, Stan Zammit and colleagues extended the original study in three ways. First, they used data from the Swedish National Hospital Discharge Register to 1996, which identified almost twice as many (362) cases of hospitalised schizophrenia as their previous study. Second, they expanded the outcomes to include bipolar affective disorder, severe depression and other psychoses. Third, they used a survival analysis (Cox regression) which took account of censoring (see page 53), although, finding that this did not substantially alter the results, they reported odds ratios obtained using logistic regression. For an explanation of survival analysis, Cox regression and logistic regression, see pages 52–56.

The association between test scores and schizophrenia was very similar to that seen in the earlier study, and again, mechanical ability was the strongest predictor. 'Other psychoses' followed a similar pattern. Severe depression was also associated with poor performance, although the magnitude of the association was smaller than for schizophrenia. There was no association between cognitive test score and risk for bipolar disorder.

Gunnell et al., 2002

David Gunnell and colleagues (Gunnell et al., 2002) performed a similar study, using a larger dataset but a shorter follow-up. The cohort comprised around 200,000 males who were conscripted between 1990 and 1997, with follow-up using the National Hospital Discharge Register to the end of 1997 to identify 60 cases of schizophrenia and 92 of non-affective, non-schizophrenic psychosis. Since subjects were only followed for a mean of 5 years from age 18, there was a strong bias towards early-onset cases. Through linkage to the Swedish Medial Birth Register, the authors were able to control for birthweight, birth length, gestational age, Apgar score, maternal age and parity, as well as parental education level. They used a survival analysis (Cox proportional hazards).

Like the previous studies, poor scores strongly predicted schizophrenia, and to a lesser extent, other non-affective psychoses. There was no evidence of confounding by pregnancy or birth variables. Of the cognitive domains, the technical and logic scores were the strongest predictors of schizophrenia, but all domains were predictive. There was also evidence that being in the lowest category conferred a greater risk than one would have expected.

A fascinating finding was that the strongest predictor of both schizophrenia and non-affective psychosis, which also showed the greatest discrimination between schizophrenia and other non-affective psychoses, was a subjective score indicating suitability for officer status, based on a structured interview by a psychologist. This suggests that the typical pre-schizophrenia deficit may be better captured by a subjective assessment incorporating a range of global cognitive and social abilities rather than any specific test.

NATIONAL COLLABORATIVE PERINATAL PROJECT

The National Collaborative Perinatal Project is an American birth cohort from 1959 to 1966 conducted at multiple sites. The sample underwent neuropsychological testing using the Stanford–Binet IQ test at ages 4 and the Wechsler Intelligence Scale for Children at age 7, and were assessed for psychotic symptoms at a mean age of 23.

Bill Kremen and colleagues published a study in 1998 based on data from the Rhode Island sample of the project (Kremen et al., 1998). Although only four children had developed schizophrenia, 18 (3%) had 'definite or probable' psychotic symptoms. Children with the greatest (top 10%) decline in IQ between ages 4 and 7 had around a sevenfold increased risk of psychotic or probable psychotic symptoms at age 23 (confidence interval not presented), and decline was a better predictor of psychosis than raw score at either age. The association seemed specific to psychotic symptoms, and was not present for mania, depression, anxiety, antisocial personality or substance misuse. However, Ty Cannon later published data from the Philadelphia sample of the project, showing that patients who would later develop schizophrenia had global deficits at both time points but no decline between 4 and 7 (Cannon et al., 2000).

Although the small sample and 'soft' outcome measure limit the impact of these studies, their strength is their ability to model changes in IQ over time.

ISRAELI CONSCRIPT STUDIES

Davidson et al., 1999

I have previously described this study on page 23. Schizophrenic patients performed significantly worse than controls. Although unremarked by the authors, there was an excess of patients with schizophrenia in the highest two performance bands. There was no statistical test as to whether this excess was likely to be a chance finding, although a test for departure from linear trend was not significant.

As well as test scores, a variety of behavioural measures, such as social functioning, organisational ability, interest in physical activity and individual autonomy were also strongly associated with risk for schizophrenia.

Weiser et al., 2000

Michael Davidson's study was confined to males, since only males had data on behavioural measures. However, cognitive data existed for both sexes. In a separate paper, Mark Weiser compared the scores from males and females in this sample, and found that girls who would later develop schizophrenia also had a pre-morbid deficit, which was somewhat more pronounced than that of males (Weiser et al., 2000).

Reichenberg et al., 2002

Avi Reichenberg then extended the findings from the previous study in several ways (Reichenberg et al., 2002). First, the size of the sample was increased, by adding another 4 years (up to 1995) and extending follow-up by 1 year (to 1996). Second, by focusing only on cognitive tests, which were taken by both sexes, females could also be included. Third, the diagnoses were extended to include bipolar disorder and schizoaffective disorder. Fourth, the authors examined the subtests from the cognitive battery. Again, the design was a nested case–control study, this time with conventional one-to-one matching on age, sex and school. Individuals who would go on to develop schizophrenia showed significant deficits in all measures, and those individuals who would develop schizoaffective disorders showed a similar impairment, whereas patients with bipolar disorder did not differ from controls on any measure.

Reichenberg et al., 2005

In a further elaboration of this study, the authors conducted a cohort study using a survival analysis, with a larger sample (Reichenberg et al., 2005). In this study, the exposure of interest was not the actual pre-morbid performance but an estimate of pre-morbid intellectual decline, based on the discrepancy between measures of IQ at conscription (age 16–17) and scores on reading, vocabulary and spelling abilities, which were assumed to reflect IQ earlier in childhood. Children with the greatest discrepancies were more likely to develop schizophrenia. However, since this study only used measures at one time-point, it only provides suggestive evidence of decline. It is possible that these discrepancies in scores simply reflect differential deficits, rather than decline.

FINNISH STUDIES

Northern Finland 1966 Birth Cohort

I have previously described this study on page 23, in which school performance was assessed in terms of being in the expected class, and grade-point average.

As expected, being in a lower class than expected was a significant risk factor for schizophrenia (odds ratio (OR) 2.5, 95% CI 1.2 to 5.1), but surprisingly, there was an even greater effect for other psychoses and for non-psychotic mental disorders. Furthermore, among children who were in their normal class at age 16, children who would later develop schizophrenia did not differ in their grade-point average from those who would remain well. The same negative result applied to other psychoses, but children with future non-psychotic disorders did achieve significantly worse grades than the population.

It is difficult to explain why the performance of patients with non-psychotic disorders was actually worse than that of schizophrenia. However, it should be noted that these were admitted cases. Whereas almost all cases of schizophrenia are admitted at some point in the early course of disorder, this may not be the case for non-psychotic disorders, so one would expect that the few cases of non-psychotic disorders in this study were particularly severe, whereas the schizophrenia cases were probably more representative. Nevertheless, this study suggests that poor school performance may not be specific to schizophrenia.

Another unexpected finding was that boys with excellent school performance at age 16 had a fourfold increased risk of schizophrenia compared with controls. However, the numbers were small, and if two fewer cases of schizophrenia had occurred in the excellent performance group, the result would not have been statistically significant. Furthermore, the effect was completely absent in girls (Isohanni et al., 1999), and was only significant if girls were excluded.

Helsinki cohort

This was a nested case–control study within the cohort of all children born in Helsinki during a 10-year period from 1951 to 1960 (Cannon et al., 1999). The authors used the Finnish Hospital Discharge Register, Pensions Register and Free Medicines Register to identify non-hospitalised as well as hospitalised cases of schizophrenia (broadly defined as code 295 in ICD–8 and 9 (WHO, 1967, 1968)) who were born in Helsinki. School grades and teachers' ratings at ages 7–11 were identified for just under half of these children, and compared to Helsinki-born controls. Principal components analysis identified three factors from the scores: academic, non-academic and behavioural.

Again, there was an unexpectedly small difference between cases and controls. They differed only on the behavioural measure, which accounted for 11% of the total variance and loaded mainly sports and handicraft. There was no difference in class rank between cases and controls, although cases were less likely to proceed to high school at age 11.

Finnish conscript study

This study used a similar design as the Swedish and Israeli conscript studies (Tiihonen et al., 2005). Of all males born from 1962 to 1967, the 195,000 who served in the Finnish army between 1982 and 1987 (87%), were tested at mean age 20 and followed using the Finnish Hospital Discharge Register until the end of 1991, when they were aged 24–29.

Poor performance on a test of visuospatial reasoning predicted higher risks of schizophrenia and bipolar disorder. Arithmetic reasoning and verbal reasoning do not appear to have predicted either disorder from the data presented – none of the performance categories significantly differed from the reference category, but the odds ratios for trend were not given.

I have some concerns with the analysis of this study. In particular, the authors claim that higher scores in arithmetic ability are associated with increased risks of bipolar disorder. However, the apparent trend is observed only after adjusting for performance in the other two cognitive domains. Given that the other two domains show strong trends in the opposite direction, controlling for them produces an apparent trend despite the absence of any real association between arithmetic ability and risk for bipolar disorder. When one examines the raw scores, there is no evidence that higher scores are associated with bipolar disorder – if anything, they are somewhat protective against bipolar, although none of the performance categories differ from the reference category.

DUNEDIN COHORT

The Dunedin cohort has been described on page 24. Mary Cannon and colleagues conducted a nested case–control study within this cohort (Cannon et al., 2002b). There was a marked and significant difference between schizophreniform disorder and controls for both IQ and receptive (but not expressive) language at ages 3, 5, 7, 9 and 11, whereas those with future mania or anxiety or depressive disorders did not differ from controls. Similar patterns were observed for non-cognitive indicators of development, including motor skills and neurological signs – indeed, children with future mania had significantly better motor development than controls. These associations did not change after adjusting for obstetric complications. Children who reported psychotic symptoms at age 11 had significantly lower IQ and receptive language development in the first decade of life than controls. As previously reported, children who went on to develop mania had better cognitive performance than controls, although numbers were small.

COPENHAGEN SAMPLE

In another register study, similar in design to the other Scandinavian studies, Osler and colleagues (2007) examined the influence of cognitive function at ages 12 and 18 on risk for hospital admission for schizophrenia or bipolar disorder in 6923 members of a birth cohort who had cognitive data at both time-points. Those with schizophrenia or schizophrenia-spectrum disorder were combined into one group (n=133), and showed poor pre-morbid cognitive function and also cognitive decline. There were too few cases of bipolar disorder for a meaningful analysis.

SUMMARY AND CONCLUSIONS

It is now beyond question that schizophrenia is associated with pre-morbid cognitive deficits. Most studies have found a generalised deficit affecting most or all domains, with no clear pattern of differential deficits. The timing of these deficits is less clear, with the British, Israeli, Danish and Rhode Island studies suggesting that the deficits become more extreme with time, but the New Zealand and Philadelphia studies demonstrating deficits from as early as age 3, with no evidence of decline.

Fewer studies have examined bipolar disorder, and those that have are less easy to interpret, because of the nosological inconsistencies between classification systems, and the consequent tendency to combine bipolar disorder with other disorders. However, the weight of evidence favours the view that there is little or no deficit associated with bipolar disorder.

There seems to be some evidence from the Finnish and Israeli studies to support the hypothesis of an association between high cognitive functioning and schizophrenia, at least in males.

The two Finnish studies on school performance are unique in failing to find large deficits in children who will go on to develop schizophrenia, although subtle differences did emerge. It seems unlikely that the relationship between pre-morbid cognitive functioning and schizophrenia would differ between Finland and the other countries studied, so the most likely explanation is that school performance, at least in Finland, does not capture these cognitive deficits. This is unexpected, since many studies have shown strong correlations between school performance and IQ (Deary et al., 2007).

Most of these studies have shown similar findings with respect to schizophrenia, but areas of uncertainty still exist: the timing of cognitive deficits in childhood, and whether there is any decline during childhood; whether there are any deficits in bipolar disorder and schizoaffective disorder; whether school performance is impaired at all in any psychotic disorder; whether high cognitive function is a risk factor for any psychotic disorders.

The role of confounders in these associations also needs to be clarified. Many of the exposures that are associated with schizophrenia are also risk factors for poor cognitive function. These include socioeconomic group, parental education level, pregnancy and birth complications or abnormalities (Seidman et al., 2000; Richards et al., 2001; Matte et al., 2001), season of birth (Lawlor et al., 2006), parental (particularly paternal) age at birth (Malaspina et al., 2005), and migration or minority status (Gonzalez, 2003; Perreira et al., 2006). Some studies have controlled for some of these confounders, but none has been able to control for all simultaneously.

CHAPTER FOUR

The study of pre-morbid school performance in schizophrenia and other psychoses (SP$_3$)

AIMS AND OBJECTIVES

The ideal implementation of the scientific method is to develop a hypothesis and then design the perfect study to refute it (Popper, 1983). However, in the field of lifecourse epidemiology, it is rare to have the resources or time to design a study that can collect relevant data from scratch. The majority of data are obtained opportunistically, using pre-existing databases. It is therefore usually necessary to adopt a more pragmatic approach, in which a suitable dataset for answering a particular question is sought, perhaps with an ideal hypothesis in mind, and the exact hypothesis to be tested is decided once the limitations of the data are known.

My starting point was that I wished to investigate intellectual function as a risk marker for psychosis. Armed with a thorough knowledge of the literature, and of the current questions in the field, as summarised above, I set out to find a dataset that would enable me to further our understanding of this area. Having found a potential dataset, I would assess the potential of the data to address questions of interest in the field, and, if I believed a valuable study could be conducted, formulate specific hypotheses pertaining to those data.

In this chapter, I will begin by describing the rationale for my choice of study design, and then describe the process of identifying, obtaining and analysing a suitable dataset. I will then describe the data in detail, including important background information such as a description of the education system in Sweden.

I will also describe the process of linking and processing the data in some detail, since this process was far more complicated and time consuming than I had anticipated, and demanded rigorous attention to detail. I was struck by how easy it would be to generate inaccurate or biased data through a careless programming error, without being aware that a mistake had been made.

CHOICE OF STUDY DESIGN

Retrospective case–control study

This design would perhaps have been the easiest to conduct. In such a design, cases of schizophrenia would have been obtained through clinical contacts, and control subjects from public advertisements or from a general hospital, with group matching or individual matching for age, gender and other potential confounders. The two groups (cases and controls) would then have been compared with respect to their pre-morbid intellectual function. Siblings could have been added as a third group, to assess to what extent any decrement in pre-morbid function was shared within families.

There are two common approaches to estimating pre-morbid academic functioning in case–control studies. The first is to use a clinical estimator of pre-morbid intelligence, such as the National Adult Reading Test (Nelson, 1982), a test of familiarity with irregularly spelled words. However, the NART is probably only a good estimator of verbal intelligence, and does not correlate highly with other domains of cognitive function (Schretlen et al., 2005). Furthermore, there is some evidence that the NART performance is affected by cognitive decline in schizophrenia, as well as in other disorders, such as dementia (Tracy et al., 1996).

The second method of estimating pre-morbid cognitive function is to use educational achievement as a proxy for academic ability; for example, the number of years of study or the level of academic qualifications obtained. I have previously conducted a study using such a measure, in which patients with university degrees were identified by systematically searching case notes (MacCabe et al., 2002). The object of that study was to compare patients with high and 'normal' intellectual functioning, so the 'controls' were schizophrenic patients without a university degree.

However, even this relatively simple classification may have poor validity, because of population changes over time. The proportion of young adults obtaining a degree in the UK doubled from 15% to 30% over the 1990s alone (Higher Education Funding Council of England (HEFCE), 1999). Some or all of the increase may be due to better access to degree courses for students from less privileged backgrounds. It has also been suggested that the academic standard required for some UK qualifications, particularly GCSEs and A-levels, may have fallen over the past two decades. Whatever its cause, the problem illustrates the drawbacks of retrospectively assessing intellectual function using educational attainment, particularly in a sample with a wide age range.

I have already discussed two fundamental problems with case–control designs in Chapter 3, namely their inability to distinguish between pre-morbid and illness-related effects, and the difficulty of eliminating selection bias.

The final reason for rejecting a case–control design was that I wanted to make a substantial contribution to the academic literature. There have been countless case–control studies of cognition in schizophrenia, but only a handful of prospective cohort studies, and it is the cohort studies that have yielded the most important results with regard to pre-morbid cognitive function. It was difficult to see how a further retrospective case–control study would have greatly advanced our knowledge in this field.

Cohort study

A cohort study has the advantage that the data are collected prospectively, and are therefore not likely to be influenced by the outcome. In a traditional cohort study, a group of healthy individuals (the cohort) is identified and assessed for the exposure (in this case, some measure of intellectual functioning). The individuals are then monitored for the outcome (psychosis in this case). The analysis then compares the risks or rates for the outcome between exposed and unexposed individuals.

A traditional cohort study would have been impractical as the resources and time involved would have been very substantial. Furthermore, for a relatively rare outcome such as psychosis, a very large number of well individuals would have had to be surveyed in order to identify a sufficient number of cases for meaningful analysis.

Alternative approaches

Two alternative study designs are becoming increasingly common in modern epidemiology: the nested case–control design and the historical cohort design. Both of these approaches are therefore particularly suited to exploiting routinely collected datasets in which all exposure and outcome information is already recorded.

Nested case–control study

In a nested case–control study, cases are identified from within an existing cohort. For each case, one or more controls is selected from the cohort.

Matching can be used at this stage to ensure comparability between the cases and controls, although there is a recent movement within epidemiology to adjust for potential confounders in the analysis instead of matching for them, as this reduces the probability of overmatching and allows the effect of the confounder to be modelled (Langholz & Clayton, 1994). Cases and controls are then compared with respect to the exposure, as in a classical case–control study. As in all case–control studies, it is vital to minimise selection bias by ensuring that the cases are selected using exactly the same criteria as the controls. However, unlike traditional case–control studies, the data on exposure are collected prospectively and so are not affected by recall bias.

Historical cohort study

These studies are sometimes referred to as retrospective cohort studies, because the study is conceptually a cohort study, but conducted after the data have been collected. Historical cohort studies have most of the advantages of a traditional cohort study, in that the data on exposure are collected prospectively, without knowledge of the outcome.

Because both these alternative designs use pre-existing datasets, much larger datasets can potentially be used, and the study can be completed more quickly, than with traditional designs. However, both designs suffer from three practical drawbacks: first, the data are not usually collected with the study hypothesis in mind, so the researcher often has to use incomplete, proxy or imputed data. Second, relevant datasets, if they exist at all, can be difficult to find and access. Third, the data for these studies are not always 'owned' by a particular research group, so there is a risk that the same study, or one very similar, may already have been undertaken by another researcher; worse still, the other researcher may be working simultaneously on the same data.

Having considered the various options for study design, particularly in the light of the existing literature, it was clear that a cohort study would be preferable, and that given the time and resources available, an existing dataset would be essential. The task was therefore to find a suitable cohort. The prerequisites of the cohort were as follows:

1. standardised assessments of cognitive function or educational attainment before illness onset;
2. reliable and comprehensive follow-up information;
3. large enough to have adequate power to detect relevant differences – preferably larger than existing studies.

In addition, the following features were desirable:

4. the ability to adjust for pregnancy and birth complications, socioeconomic group and other potential confounders;
5. detailed cognitive assessments of different domains;
6. detailed clinical information such as age at onset, presence of particular symptoms and measures of disease severity.

At the time that I was planning this study (2003), birth cohorts had been used successfully in the UK (Jones and Done, 1997), the USA (Cannon et al., 2000) and New Zealand (Cannon et al., 2002b), but these had the disadvantage of being relatively small, with relatively high attrition rates. Another birth cohort study, in Finland (Isohanni et al., 1998), had been able to use national registers of routinely collected hospital data for follow-up, which gave the advantage of a low attrition rate. Unfortunately, this strategy would not have been possible in most countries, such as the UK, where such registers do not exist. In any case, I did not know of the existence of any other birth cohorts that might have been useable for my purposes.

A second possibility was the use of army conscription registers. Arguably the largest and most impressive studies to date had used conscription registers in Sweden and Israel, including a study by one of my supervisors, Anthony David (David et al., 1997). These studies made use of standardised cognitive tests at conscription, which were linked to hospital or psychiatric registers to detect cases of psychosis in the entire population with nearly universal coverage. These studies were considered the 'gold standard' in the field and served as a model in my search for a cohort.

IDENTIFYING A SWEDISH DATASET

Fortunately, my other supervisor, Robin Murray, had a pre-existing collaboration with Christina Hultman, a psychiatric epidemiologist at the Department of Medical Epidemiology and Biostatistics at the Karolinska Institutet in Stockholm. Through Dr Hultman, and her colleague, Mats Lambe, I discovered the existence of the Swedish School Register.

This register, described in detail below, contains school grades for all children finishing compulsory school at a mean age of 16, for around 1.2 million individuals.

The use of school records was particularly attractive for several reasons.

1. School records had been used in two Finnish studies (Isohanni et al., 1998; Cannon et al., 1999), and had yielded some unexpected results. In both studies, overall school performance appeared to have little or no bearing on subsequent risk for schizophrenia. This was in direct contrast to other studies, which had used cognitive tests as a measure

of pre-morbid functioning. These results were difficult to explain, and it was clear that further research on school performance as a predictor of psychosis was important.

2. School performance is arguably a better measure of functional ability than cognitive tests. It is a 'real-life' measure, which is associated with occupational function. Furthermore, success at school is a test of sustained effort rather than a 'snapshot' of ability on the day of testing.

3. School performance is available for almost the entire population of Sweden, including many pupils with special educational needs. Formal cognitive testing is rarely performed on such a large scale. The only example, to my knowledge, of near-universal cognitive testing, is at army conscription in countries including Sweden, Finland and Israel. However, such tests are normally confined to males, and typically exclude individuals who are excused army service; a group that is likely to contain an excess of individuals who go on to develop psychosis.

4. If the identification of children with poor cognitive function in adolescence were found to be a useful way of identifying individuals who go on to develop psychosis, it could probably be achieved more easily by using school grades than by using formal cognitive testing.

5. Information on separate school subjects was available, allowing analysis of specific subjects as risk factors for psychosis; analogous to using specific cognitive tests rather than overall intelligence.

However, school records have certain disadvantages compared with cognitive tests.

1. They are usually less standardised, although in the case of the Swedish school records, considerable efforts are made to ensure uniformity of grading nationwide, as I will describe below.

2. They are not designed to test specific cognitive functions, although it is worth noting that most routinely administered cognitive tests used in previous studies of this type are not designed to test specific brain regions (such as the frontal lobe) – they generally test broad categories of ability such as mechanical knowledge or verbal abilities.

Power calculation

Before embarking on a study it is important to establish whether the data will have the statistical power to show a clinically important effect, if such an effect is present. In most cases this involves defining the minimum effect that would be considered clinically significant, and then calculating the minimum sample size needed to demonstrate such an effect statistically.

I conducted the sample size calculation using the methods of Hsieh and Lavori (2000). In order to calculate the sample size required, certain assumptions were necessary, some of which can be made using the results of previous studies and others of which are to some extent arbitrary.

I defined the effect measure for the study as the hazard ratio for psychosis for an increase in grade-point average of one Z-score. A Z-score is equal to one standard deviation. A standard deviation is the average amount that members of a population deviate from the mean, so a Z-score represents the number of standard deviations from the mean. The use of Z-scores is common in studies of cognitive function, because it allows studies that were measured using different scales to be compared using a standardised score. For example, an increase in height of one inch is obviously different from an increase in one centimetre, whereas an increase in height of 1Z will be the same height difference (equating to around 2.8 inches, or 7 cm, for American males), regardless of whether the heights were originally measured in inches or centimetres.

I set the threshold to a hazard ratio of 0.8. A hazard ratio of 0.8 would mean that for every increase in grade-point average of 1Z, the risk for psychosis would be multiplied by 0.8, or reduced by 20%. In other words, if an increase in grade-point average of one standard deviation conferred a reduction in risk of psychosis of 20% or more, I would consider this a clinically important effect.

In the Cox proportional hazards model, the uncensored observations do not contribute to the power (Hsieh & Lavori, 2000). Therefore, the sample size calculation gives the number of failures (in this case, people developing psychosis) that will be needed to show a given effect. My calculation showed that the number of failures required to have 80% power to demonstrate an effect equating to a hazard ratio of 0.8 for a change of 1Z in the exposure would be 158. Allowing for censoring of 5% through death or migration, we would need 166 future cases of schizophrenia to be in the sample. McGrath and colleagues (2004), in their meta-analysis of the incidence of schizophrenia, showed that the median incidence was 15.2 per 100,000 years. Assuming this incidence, we would have to follow a cohort for $(166/(15.2/100000)) = 1,092,105$ person-years. From what I knew of the sample, this seemed easily attainable.[1]

---

1 Our eventual sample comfortably exceeded this for schizophrenia and bipolar disorder: 715,398 subjects were followed for 6,783,520 person-years, yielding 493 cases of schizophrenia, and 278 of bipolar disorder. However, there were only 94 cases of schizoaffective disorder, meaning that the study was not sufficiently powerful to detect an effect of the magnitude specified above; in the event the effects were also greater than predicted.

BACKGROUND INFORMATION ON THE DATA

Swedish Population Registries

History

The population registries in Sweden are a unique resource. Sweden and Finland (which was under Swedish rule until 1809) have had a national system of population registration since 1749, and are probably the only countries that possess continuous records of their population so far back in time. The data were originally collected and administered by the Church, but are now administered by a central government-based agency, *Statistiska Centralbyrån*. Initially, the main focus was on collecting population statistics for taxation purposes, but, over time, the registers have come to be valued as a resource for research, particularly in the medical and social sciences. The information in most of the registers was computerised during the 1960s.

The personnummer

A crucial development was the introduction of a personal identification number (Swedish: *personnummer*) in 1947. The personal identity number consists of 10 digits. The first six digits correspond to the person's birthday, in YYMMDD form. The seventh to ninth are a serial number, with odd numbers assigned to men, and even numbers to women. The tenth digit is a check digit, whose value is computed from the values of the other digits. Thus, 90% of transcription errors will result in the check digit failing to correspond with the remaining digits. This allows automatic error detection at the data entry stage. The *personnummer* is attached to almost all registries in Sweden. It can therefore be used to link data from disparate sources.

Extent of coverage

It is a legal requirement for anyone resident in Sweden for more than 3 months to be registered with the authorities and be issued with a *personnummer*. It is almost impossible to be resident in Sweden without being registered. Any contact with the educational, medical, banking, social welfare or other services will automatically lead to registration. There are several strong disincentives to remaining unregistered, as access to benefits, education, health care, subsidised childcare and many other services depend on having a *personnummer*.

Organisation of population databases in Sweden

The organisation responsible for the maintenance and administration of the majority of Swedish population statistics is Statistiska Centralbyrån, which translates as 'Central Office of Statistics' although the organisation refers to itself in English as Statistics Sweden.

Datasets are compiled by Statistics Sweden on receipt of a written request, from an appropriate source such as a university department. Data from the different population registers must be linked electronically using the *personnummer*. However, the anonymity of the data must be preserved to prevent unauthorised use of the data. The solution to this problem is to use a 'running number', or *löpnummer*, for register linkage. The *person-nummer* is converted to a *löpnummer* using a unique key, which applies only to that study. All the datasets requested for a particular study use the same key, so the *löpnummer* can be used by the researchers to link the registers together. The registers are delivered as separate files (frequently more than one data file per register) all of which use compatible *löpnummers*.

Following delivery of a set of data, the researchers are given a grace period of 3 months in which to link and perform initial analyses of the data and to identify any problems with the data, or additional data that are needed. After this period has elapsed, the key used in the study is destroyed, meaning that the link between *löpnummers* and *personnummers* is permanently broken. The system of using *löpnummers* that are not compatible between studies ensures that researchers can only link together datasets requested for the same study, and cannot compile their own population databases by unauthorised linkage of data from different studies.

The Centre for Epidemiology at the National Board of Health and Welfare is responsible for keeping health-related statistics in Sweden. Two of the databases used in this study (the Medical Birth Register and the Hospital Discharge Register) were provided by this organisation, who co-ordinated with Statistics Sweden to ensure that the same key was used to convert *pesonnummers* to *löpnummers*.

Swedish education system

Education in Sweden is free of charge and compulsory between the ages of 7 and 16. The school year runs from August to June, and children are assigned to their class according to their calendar year of birth. All children therefore begin school during the calendar year of their seventh birthday and finish their compulsory schooling in June of the year in which they turn 16, thus completing their compulsory education at a mean age of almost exactly 16.0.

Approximately 100,000 pupils complete their compulsory school each year. This includes those attending the standard compulsory school (*grundskolan*), Sami school (*sameskolan*) (for Sami-speaking children in the far north of Sweden), independent compulsory schools, special schools (*specialskolan*) for children with hearing, vision or speech disabilities, and compulsory school for the learning disabled (*särskolan*),

Sami school

There are only around 150 pupils enrolled in the Sami school. Sami school is available only in years 1–6 (of 9), after which Sami children join their peers in mainstream compulsory school.

Physical and sensory disabilities

The majority of pupils with physical (including sensory) disabilities attend mainstream compulsory school. For children who need more specialised teaching, there are also eight special schools for a total of around 800 pupils, which should, as far as possible, provide equivalent education to that offered in the compulsory schools. The majority of these special schools are for pupils with hearing impairments.

Learning disability

There is a strong focus on inclusion of learning disabled children in compulsory school, where they either follow the standard curriculum, with extra support, or may be enrolled in special classes for the learning disabled. Between 1 and 2% of Swedish pupils attend schools catering exclusively for learning disabilities (Lundh, 2003).

Independent schools

Prior to 1992, less than 1% of Swedish children attended private schools. However, a change in legislation in 1992 encouraged the expansion of this sector, and it had grown to around 5% by 1998 (the latest year of graduation from compulsory school in this study). Independent schools are obliged to follow the same national curriculum and assessments as the state-funded compulsory schools.

Compulsory schools

Around 98% of pupils in compulsory school attend schools run by the municipalities, usually in their local area. Parents can, however, choose to let their children attend a school outside the home municipality. All compulsory schooling is co-educational.

Swedish, English and mathematics occupy a prominent position in compulsory school. English and mathematics are streamed, with pupils being allocated to the upper or lower stream according to ability. For each of these subjects, about two-thirds of pupils are allocated to the upper stream. There is no streaming for any of the other school subjects.

The sciences (biology, physics, chemistry and technology) are usually taught and examined separately, but may be taught and examined together in a minority of schools. The same applies to four subjects that are termed 'social sciences' in Sweden, namely geography, history, religion and civics (the comparative study of models of national government). The decision as to whether the sciences and social sciences should be examined separately or together is taken at the level of the local authority, and is not dependent on the academic performance of the school or pupil.

All students study a third language (in addition to English and Swedish), which may be their mother tongue, additional English or Swedish, or another foreign language such as Spanish. An additional optional subject may also be offered as a pupil or school option. There is a standard national syllabus for all school subjects. Table 4.1 shows the approximate number of hours devoted to each subject.

TABLE 4.1

Timetable for curriculum. Stipulates the teaching hours for subjects or groups of subjects over the 9 years of compulsory school. These figures are for 1998. Some school subjects may have received slightly more or less teaching during the study period (1988–97) but any differences are likely to be small

Subject	Minimum hours as of 1 Jan 1998
Art	230
Domestic science	118
Sports and health education	500
Music	230
Handicraft	330
Swedish	1490
English	480
Mathematics	900
Geography, history, religion, civics	885
Biology, physics, chemistry, technology	800
Foreign language	320
Pupils' choice	382
Total	6665

Assessment

Peer-referencing versus criterion-referencing

Most educational assessments use one of two broad types of scoring systems. These are referred to as peer-referencing and criterion-referencing.

In a peer-referenced (also called norm-referenced) test, the performance of each individual is compared with that of his peers, or with a sample thereof. Typically, the raw scores of a test are ranked, and a pupil's grade reflects his position in the ranking. For example, the top 5% might be awarded grade A, the next 15% grade B, and so on. The alternative is a criterion-referenced system, in which a set of targets is defined *a priori*, and pupils' work is graded according to whether it satisfies these criteria.

Each system has its advantages, but in my view, a peer-referenced system is more suitable for assessing pre-morbid abilities, for the following reasons.

1. Because they are calculated from ranks, the grades from a peer-referenced system approximate a normal distribution, even if the underlying raw scores that were used to construct them are not normally distributed. This statistical property makes them easy to manipulate and analyse. For example, their normal distribution allows the calculation of Z-scores, discussed further below.
2. Most standardized tests of intelligence and cognitive function, such as the Wechsler Adult Intelligence Scale (Wechsler, 1997), are peer-referenced, so are more easily compared with other peer-referenced measures than with criterion-referenced tests.
3. Since the same proportion of grades is awarded each year, there is no drift over time in overall grades. Criterion-referenced assessments typically show 'grade inflation': improvements from year to year, which may be related to increasing familiarity of teachers with the test, or changes in the criteria, rather than genuine changes in the ability of the population. Such changes would need to be taken into account, complicating the analysis.

The method of assessment in Swedish schools was peer-referenced until 1997. The system was specifically designed to provide a standardised measure of overall performance throughout the nation, as these scores were used to determine eligibility to upper secondary school. The curriculum was entirely replaced in a rolling programme starting in 1994, and the assessment was replaced by the current, criterion-referenced system, in 1998. The descriptions in this book refer only to the education system up to 1998, as I did not use any grades from the new criterion-referenced system.

Grading system

At the end of the final year of compulsory education, all children sat examinations in all school subjects. During the time relevant to the study (1988–97), grades were awarded on a five-grade scale for the last 2 years of compulsory schooling (this was replaced by a four-grade system in 1998, which I did not use in this study). The grades given are numbered one to five, but since numerical grades can be ambiguous, I will refer to them by letters throughout the rest of the book: 'A' denoting the best performance, and 'E' the worst. The final grade in each subject, marking the end of compulsory education, is very important to the pupils, as it determines the stream to which they will be allocated in upper secondary classes, which, although not compulsory, are attended by around 98% of pupils.

Peer-referencing of grades

Swedish and mathematics were examined by the same examination nationally. Grades were awarded to pupils according to the scheme shown in Table 4.2, which was intended to give a normal distribution of scores, with a mean of 3 (C grade) and a standard deviation of 1.

TABLE 4.2
Intended distribution of grades in nationally standardised subjects

Grade	A	B	C	D	E
Points	5	4	3	2	1
Proportion of pupils awarded (%)	7	24	38	24	7

For the other subjects, the examination papers were set at local level. The results from the nationally standardised tests were used to determine the relative performance of each class within the country.

The rank of the class within the country determined the number of grades at each level (A, B, C. . .) that could be awarded by the teacher in all the other subjects. For example, a class that performed below average on the standardised tests would be allocated fewer A and B grades and more D and E grades than an average class. Conversely, a class that performed well in the standardised tests would be allocated more A grades and fewer E grades.

For each school subject, the teachers then allocated the available grades to the pupils in each class. The allocation of grades for each school subject was based almost entirely on the pupils' scores in the examination for that subject. However, teachers had limited power to adjust a pupil's grade up or down by one point in exceptional circumstances. For example, a pupil's grade might be increased if he had suffered a bereavement or been ill at the time of the examinations, or reduced if he was found to have cheated.

This flexibility may have tempted some teachers to attempt to manipulate their overall results so as to raise the overall grades of their pupils. To minimise any such manipulation of scores, teachers were not allowed to make adjustments to the grades within their class that would change the class mean for that subject by more than 0.2 grades.

Following the allocation of grades in each subject, a grade-point average (*medelbetyg*) was then calculated for each pupil. The original purpose of this grade was to stream pupils for upper secondary education. Optional subjects were counted if this would increase the pupil's grade, but not otherwise. The grade-point average had a possible range of one to five (five representing A grades in every subject) and was expressed to the nearest 0.1. A score of zero was awarded if a pupil was absent from the exams or from school.

FINALISING THE STUDY DESIGN

On the basis of the above information, I decided to conduct a population-based study with educational attainment at age 16 as the exposure and admission for schizophrenia, schizoaffective disorder, bipolar affective disorder or other psychoses as the outcome. Having made this decision, it was clear that many other aspects of the study design, including which variables could be included as confounders, would largely be determined by the information that could be obtained by linking to other registers.

The only other constraint was computer processing power, since the more elaborate the dataset and analysis, the greater the computing power needed. My Swedish colleagues warned me that complicated analyses such as multi-level models on datasets of this size could take several days to run, with a high chance of 'crashing' the computer. Considering the number of analyses that would be conducted, particularly while exploring the effects of confounders, and the fact that I would have to conduct all analyses during short visits to Stockholm, such delays would make the study unworkable.

These problems of computer power would be largely a function of the number of subjects included in the analysis. Although a cohort study is scientifically preferable, changing to a nested case–control study would drastically reduce the number of subjects with only a small reduction in precision. I therefore decided to attempt to conduct a cohort study, reverting to a nested case–control study if this proved unworkable.

CHOICE OF STATISTICAL DESIGN

Logistic regression

Logistic regression is frequently used in the analysis of cohort studies in which the outcome is a binary variable, such as developing a disease or not. Logistic regression uses maximum likelihood theory to model the odds of developing the disorder in relation to a set of explanatory variables. However, logistic regression has two drawbacks when analysing cohort studies. The first is that logistic regression calculates the odds ratio, but the measure of interest in a cohort study is usually the risk ratio or rate ratio. The odds ratio is only an approximation of the risk or rate ratio, and is always greater in magnitude. However, for rare outcomes, such as schizophrenia and bipolar disorder, the odds ratio and risk ratio are numerically similar enough to be considered equivalent.

The second drawback of logistic regression is that it does not take into account time exposed. Logistic regression can be appropriate in cohort studies where all subjects are followed up for the same amount of time, since the risk of developing the disease is then equivalent to the proportion of subjects who have developed the disease by the end of follow-up.

However, in most cohort studies, including the present study, not all subjects are followed for the same amount of time. In the current study, it would be necessary to follow up the subjects as close to the present day as possible, but the subjects would have received their grades at different times, so older individuals would have been at risk for schizophrenia for longer than younger ones. Furthermore, individuals who had developed psychosis, died or emigrated (thus lost to follow-up) would no longer be at risk for psychosis for the purposes of the study. This time dependence should be taken into account in the analysis.

Survival analysis

Survival analysis refers to a group of statistical techniques that were originally applied to clinical trials in terminal illnesses (hence the name), but are now widely used in cohort studies with non-fatal outcomes.

The basic data required for any survival analysis are the dates of the start and end of the time that the individual is considered at risk of developing the outcome, and the status of each individual at the end of the time at risk. The date of entry is usually the start of the follow-up period. The exit date is the date at which the individual either develops the disorder or is censored. Censoring refers to the time after which the subject is no longer at risk. Subjects who die or are lost to follow-up (for example by emigrating) are censored before the study is completed – the remainder are censored on reaching the end of the follow-up period.

Classical survival analysis

The number of new disease events, divided by the total number of person-years at risk, is the incidence rate of the disease. The incidence rate ratio for a given exposure is calculated by dividing the incidence rate of individuals in the exposed group by the incidence rate in the comparison group. In the current study, the exposed group might be individuals who score below a certain threshold in their school grades, and the comparison group might be children with average performance.

The main drawback of this classical approach is that the only way to control for potential confounders is to stratify on each confounder and calculate stratum-specific rate ratios for the exposure variable at each level of the confounder variable. These stratum-specific rate ratios can then be combined using the method of Mantel and Haenszel (1959). However the number of strata becomes unworkable when more than two or three confounding variables have to be taken into account simultaneously. Furthermore, if more than one explanatory variable is of interest (e.g. different levels of scholastic achievement), a separate analysis has to be performed for each, since the procedure does not allow for the simultaneous estimation of different exposure effects.

Both of these drawbacks can be overcome by using a regression procedure. There are two commonly used regression techniques for the analysis of survival data, named after their originators, Poisson and Cox.

Poisson regression

In Poisson regression, the follow-up time (or the individuals' age) is divided into bands, and the dataset is expanded so that each observation corresponds, not to an individual, but to a unit of person-time at risk, such as a person-year of follow-up (Loomis et al., 2005). The incidence rate in each time band can then be calculated, and combined to form an overall, time- or age-adjusted rate.

Cox's proportional hazards model

Cox's proportional hazards model can be viewed as an extension of the Poisson model described above. In the Cox model, the time bands are divided into the smallest units possible, defined by the events themselves (i.e. incident cases of disease in a cohort). Thus, whereas Poisson regression uses relatively large time bands of fixed width, each containing a variable number of events, each time band in Cox's regression contains only one event, but the width of the bands can vary.

Cox regression gives a hazard ratio, which is an estimate of the ratio of the instantaneous event rate between two groups at any given time-point during the follow-up period. This is numerically close to the incidence rate ratio, and is always closer than the odds ratio (Callas et al., 1994). An important assumption in Cox regression is that the hazard ratio between the two groups being compared does not change systematically over time: the so-called proportional hazards assumption. In the current study, the proportional hazards assumption would be that the impact of school performance on developing psychosis does not change over time.

Which regression method to use?

Empirical studies have demonstrated that in most cohort studies, Cox and Poisson models give very similar results, whereas logistic regression, although widely used, may give misleading results (Callas et al., 1998), as it does not take into account the time-dependent nature of cohort studies.

Cox has some advantages over Poisson regression. First, the relationship between rate and time is modelled as finely as possible. Second, there are computational advantages, as the dataset does not need to be expanded. However, it has some disadvantages as well. First, because of the proportional hazards assumption, important time-dependent changes in hazard ratio can easily be overlooked. Second, it is difficult to take into account data that are not independent. Although the results will not be presented in this book, I designed the dataset to allow the identification of siblings for future studies investigating whether any deficits operated at the family or individual level. It would therefore be appropriate to use a model that allows for the fact that the school performance will vary less within families than between families. There are well-developed methods for dealing with such data under Poisson regression, but frailty models under the Cox model are less well developed, frequently have problems such as failure to converge, and are generally unworkable on large datasets.

My conclusions were that Cox or Poisson models would be equally suitable, but that I should check that the results were similar using both. I would preferentially use Poisson regression, to allow the results to be comparable to any analyses I would subsequently undertake using data from siblings.

REGISTERS USED IN THE STUDY

During the course of my investigations, I examined the data from several registers, and I will now describe the registers that I selected for inclusion in the study.

National School Register

The Swedish National School Register contains the individual school grades and the grade-point average for all pupils graduating from class 9, the final year of compulsory education described above, since 1988. The normal graduation age was 16 years, so the 1972 birth cohort was the first to be covered by this register. The grading system described above was in use for the first 9 years of the register's existence, between 1988 and 1997, after which it was replaced by a new, criterion-referenced system. The new system was not used in this study so it will not be considered further. Pupils with learning disabilities were included in the register if they attended mainstream compulsory school. Pupils of special schools for children with hearing impairment were probably not included, although I have been unable to obtain reliable information on this. In any case, these children constituted less than 0.1% of all children. Independent schools, which provided around 1% of compulsory education in Sweden in 1992, were included in the register from 1993 onwards.

It was important to identify a valid measure of general ability for most of the main analyses. Ideally, this measure should be standardised and comparable over the entire sample, and should reflect general ability rather than specific skills.

I initially considered using the results from a single subject, or a small group of core subjects. The subjects of Swedish or mathematics, since they were compulsory, comprised a large part of the curriculum, and were examined using nationally standardised tests. However, mathematics was streamed, and there was no agreed method of comparing the scores of the pupils from higher and lower streams (Sundin, personal communication, 2005).

Swedish was examined in a uniform way nationally, but the amount of teaching in Swedish was not uniform. Immigrants had the option to study their native language as their first, and Swedish as their second, language. I decided to exclude immigrants from the analysis (discussed below), negating this problem. However, there were two further difficulties with using Swedish. First, it was specifically related to language skills, so its utility as a measure of general ability was questionable. Second, like all single subjects, the measurement scale was relatively crude, with only five levels (A–E grades). I therefore chose to use grade-point average as the measure of general ability.

The data available from the register are shown in Table 4.3.

Hospital Discharge Register (HDR) 1990–2002

Data on hospital episodes in Sweden have been collected for the past hundred years. By 1983, 20 of the 26 county councils in Sweden reported all inpatient care to the Hospital Discharge Register (HDR) and in 1984, reporting to HDR was made compulsory for all hospitals. From 1987 the HDR covers all public, inpatient care in Sweden. Private health care, especially inpatient care of psychotic disorders, was very rare in Sweden during the study period.

There are four different types of information in the Hospital Discharge Register, listed in Table 4.4.

TABLE 4.3
Data available in the School Register

Variable	Comment
Personnummer	
Birth year, month	
Sex	
Nationality	
Year left school	
Childcare	
Art	
English	
English, common	Lower stream
English, special	Upper stream
Home economics	
Mother tongue	
Sports	
Mathematics	
Mathematics, common	Lower stream
Mathematics, special	Upper stream
Music	
Combined science	
Biology	
Physics	
Chemistry	
Engineering	
Combined humanities	
Geography	
History	
Religious studies	
Civics	The study of comparative government, culture and society
Handicrafts	
Swedish	
Swedish as a foreign language	
Medelbetyg	Grade-point average
Number of missing grades	
Reason for missing grades	(Non-attendance in almost all cases)

Reporting procedures

Information to HDR is delivered once a year from each of the county councils in Sweden. Each discharge during that year corresponds to one record. The *International Classification of Diseases* version 9 (ICD–9) was used from 1987 to 1996, and ICD–10 from 1997 on (WHO, 1978, 1992).

TABLE 4.4
Information in the Hospital Discharge Register

Type of data	Variable
Patient data	Personnummer
	Age
	Sex
	Place of residence
Data on the hospital	County council
	Hospital name
	Department
Administrative data	Date of discharge
	Length of stay
	Emergency or elective admission
Medical data	Primary diagnosis
	Secondary diagnoses (up to 8)
	Surgical procedures

Quality of data and underreporting in the HDR

The rapid changes of hospital organisation in Sweden make estimations of underreporting hard to make. The total number of missed discharges for acute inpatient episodes for the period 1987–1991 has been estimated to be less than 2% (Statistiska Centralbyrån, 2003). The number of discharges in 2003 with missing *personnummer* and missing main diagnosis were 0.7 and 0.9% respectively overall. However, for psychiatric care, around 8% of patients had a missing diagnosis (Vaittinen, 2003).

Medical Birth Register (MBR) 1973–1987

The Swedish Medical Birth Registry was established in 1973 and includes over 99% of all births in Sweden (Cnattingius et al., 1990). The purpose of the register is to compile information on pregnancy, delivery and the health of the neonate.

During the period relevant to this research (1973–1982), the register was constructed from standardised documents prepared by clerks at obstetric clinics, which summarised the contents of the medical records for each patient on a standard form. Standardised medical records and Medical Birth Reports were used throughout Sweden (with the exception of one county, which had very minor differences). Table 4.5 shows the data that were present from 1973–1982.

All diagnoses were classified according to the Swedish version of the ICD–8 (WHO, 1967).

TABLE 4.5
Summary of information available from the Medical Birth Register

Type of data	Variable
Identification of patient	maternal *personnummer*
	infant *personnummer*
	maternal place of residence (parish) at delivery
	delivery hospital.
Social factors	cohabitation/marital status
	parents' nationality
	mother's country/county of birth
Maternal history	previous pregnancies
	induced abortions (–1981)
	spontaneous abortions
	stillbirths
	live births
	perinatal deaths
Pregnancy	date of last menstrual period
	disorders at first visit to antenatal clinic (psychiatric
	disorders not reliably recorded)
Delivery	date of admission to delivery unit
	pregnancy duration (weeks, days)
	presentation of infant (e.g. cephalic, breech)
	delivery diagnoses
	more on delivery: caesarean, forceps, vacuum extraction,
	other procedures
	analgesia, anaesthesia with specification
Infant	date and time of birth
	stillborn/live-born
	date of death, underlying cause of death
	sex
	birthweight
	birth length
	head circumference
	multiple birth, inc. number
	Apgar score at 1, 5, 10 minutes
	infant diagnoses
	operations and other treatments of infant

Multi-Generation Register (MGR) 2002

The Swedish Multi-Generation Register lists every individual who was born between 1932 and 2002, and was resident in Sweden at any time between 1961 and 2002. For each of these index individuals, the register lists his country of birth, and the *personnummer*s of his/her biological or adoptive parents. Coverage is claimed to be 100% for index individuals living in Sweden since 1998, but not all these individuals have data on their parents. The proportion with data on parents was around 85% per parent for children born in 1973, increasing to over 95% for those born in 1983 (Öhman, 2005).

Total Population Register (TPR)

This register is administered by the tax authorities, and is a record of every person living in Sweden at any one time. Data on country of origin, citizenship, deaths and emigrations and data from the Censuses and the Education Register are all available via links from the TPR.

The 1980 and 1990 Censuses

The Swedish Population and Housing Censuses of 1980 and 1990 were based on a questionnaire that included items about household size, type of housing, employment, occupation, and income. Socioeconomic status was classified into six categories: (1) blue collar, unskilled; (2) blue collar, skilled; (3) white collar (lower); (4) white collar (middle); (5) white collar (higher); (6) company owner/self-employed.

The Education Register

The Education Register (which should not be confused with the National School Register) records the educational attainment for all 16- to 74-year-olds registered in Sweden, and is updated once a year. Education is recorded as five levels: (1) compulsory school only (9 years); (2) upper secondary school (2 years); (3) upper secondary school (3 years); (4) higher education (<3 years); and (5) higher education (≥3 years). The register uses the censuses of 1970 and 1990 as its base, and data are added each year from higher educational institutions. A validation in 1990 showed that the highest level of formal education is correctly reported in 83% (Cnattingius et al., 1990), but the more recent addition of data from higher education registers from 1988 onwards should have improved this figure.

CONSTRUCTING THE DATABASE

Obtaining the dataset

Source of the datasets

The data had to be ordered from two separate organisations. The Medical Birth Register and Hospital Discharge Register were administered by the Centre for Epidemiology (EpC) at the National Board of Health and Welfare, whereas the other databases were kept by Statistics Sweden. To preserve confidentiality, the datasets would be supplied with a temporary 'running number' (Swedish: löpnummer) in place of the personnummer, as explained above. The encoding of the *löpnummer* would be performed by Statistics Sweden, who would then pass the dataset, along with the key, to EpC so that linkable datasets from the Medical Birth Register and Hospital Discharge Register could be produced. The linkage procedure would be very complex, and had to be specified in detail before the data were ordered, to allow these organisations to collaborate in producing datasets that could be linked successfully. My Swedish collaborators, particularly Mats Lambe, assisted me greatly with this step. We devised the following broad study plan, the details of which would be modified later.

Sampling frame

The sampling frame was initially defined as all individuals born in 1973 or later (the first year of the Medical Birth Register) recorded in the School Register from 1988 (the first year in the School Register, and the year that most children born in 1973 completed class 9) to the end of 2003.

Overview of linkage procedure

Taking the school database as the starting point, the personal identification number would be used to link to the Hospital Discharge Register to identify data on hospital admissions for psychosis. The database would also be linked to the Multi-Generation Register to retrieve the parents' *löpnummers*. These parents' *löpnummers* would be used to link to the censuses, the Total Population Register, and the Education Register, to collect data on country of birth, socioeconomic group, and parental age and education. Finally, the data from the Medical Birth Registry would then be linked in. I passed these requirements to Statistics Sweden and requested the dataset.

Structure of the dataset

Table 4.6 lists the files that I received.

Relation file

The relation file would be used only for linkage, and consisted of the index person's *löpnummer* followed by the *löpnummers* of their parents.

Parental social background

There were separate files for fathers and mothers. The data in the files are shown in Table 4.7.

TABLE 4.6
Data received from Statistics Sweden and the EpC

Filename	Explanation	Observations
Statistics Sweden		
Relation_Up197387Foraldrar	Relation file	1,753,018
Far_Up197387	Father's social background	939,389
Mor_Up197387	Mother's social background	961,475
Up197387SkolrAr8893	Index child school results 1988–1993	514,900
Up197387SkolrAr9497	Index child school results 1994–1997	392,111
Up197387SkolrAr9800	Index child school results 1998–2000	293,479
Up197387SkolrAr0103	Index child school results 2001–2003	316,947
EpC		
WORK.LAMBE_5445	Medical Birth Register 1973–1987	1,465,998
WORK.LAMBE_PAR	Hospital Discharge Register 1990–2002	49,124
Explanation files		
SUNInriktning	Key for parental education type	
SUNNiva	Key for parental education level	
FoB80_dokumentation.doc	Key for census information 1980	
FoB90_dokumentation.doc	Key for census information 1990	
Årskurs9_1988_93.xls	Explanations of grades	
Årskurs9_1994_97.xls	Explanations of grades	
Årskurs9_1998_00.xls	Explanations of grades	
Årskurs9_2001_03.xls	Explanations of grades	

TABLE 4.7
Data in Father's social background file

Variable name	English translation	Unit
LopNr_Far	Running number of biological father	
FodArMan	Birth year and month	
UtlSvBakgrundFar	Father's nationality	
AntBoHh80	No. in household in 1980	
Hustyp80	Type of house in 1980	
Upplform80	Rental or own home in 1980	
Yrke80	Occupation in 1980	
SEI80	Socioeconomic code in 1980	
MedbGrupp80	Citizenship grouping in 1980	
Sink80	Total income in 1980	100 SEK
AntBoHh90	No. in household in 1990	
Hustyp90	Type of house in 1990	
Upplform90	Rental or own home in 1990	
Yrke90	Occupation in 1990	
SEI90	Socioeconomic code in 1990	
Sink90	Total income in 1990	
MedbGrupp90	Citizenship grouping in 1990	100 SEK
Sun2000Niva	Educational level	
Sun2000Inr	Educational subject	

School Register

The School Register consisted of four files, because the set of subjects studied and the coding system had been changed three times from 1988 to 2003. The changes in 1993 and 2000 were minor re-categorisations of the optional subjects, with no change to the core subjects. However, in 1997, grade-point average was replaced by the new criterion-referenced system, which used a different scale and was not normally distributed. It was clear that the two systems could not be combined in the same analysis. Furthermore, the individuals in the earlier cohorts were of more interest, since they had been at risk of psychosis for longer. I therefore decided to focus only on the cohort who received their grades in 1988–1997.

The variables in these datasets are listed in Table 4.3 (p. 57).

Medical Birth Register

The Medical Birth Register consisted of one file for the entire cohort. The variables that were used are listed in Table 4.8.

TABLE 4.8
Variables used in Medical Birth Register

Variable name	English translation	Units
Apgar1	Apgar score at 1 minute	1–10
Apgar5	Apgar score at 5 minutes	1–10
Apgar10	Apgar score at 10 minutes	1–10
Blandf	Child's length	mm
Bord	Singleton/twin/triplet etc.	
Bordnr	Birth order within multiple birth	
Grvbs	Pregnancy length	weeks
Homf	Head circumference	mm
Mlga	Large for gestational age	
Msga	Small for gestational age	
Parabs	Parity	
Blopnm	Child's *löpnummer*	

Hospital Discharge Register

The Hospital Discharge Register consisted of one file for the entire cohort. The variables within the register are shown in Table 4.9.

Additional data on death and emigration

After delivery of the data, I realised that I had made a small error when ordering the data. In order to take into account censoring within the data, I

TABLE 4.9
Variables in Hospital Discharge Register

Variable name	English translation	Unit
Diagnos	Secondary diagnosis	ICD–9 and 10
Hdia	Main diagnosis	ICD–9 and 10
Lan	County	
Utskrivning	Discharge date	year and month
Vtid	Length of admission	days

would need data on individuals who died or emigrated during the follow-up period, and the dates of these events. I therefore requested further data on dates of deaths and emigration from Statistics Sweden. The files are listed in Table 4.10. Each file consisted of a list of *löpnummers* and dates for deaths and emigrations.

TABLE 4.10
Additional data files on death and emigration obtained from EpC

Filename	Explanation	Observations
Lambe_IndexDoda.txt	Index deaths	1,517,437
Lambe_IndexEmigrant.txt	Index permanent emigration	1,517,437
Lambe_IndexEmigrant2.txt	Index emigration including re-immigrants	1,517,437
Lambe_SyskonDoda.txt	Sibling deaths	(not used)
Lambe_SyskonEmigrant.txt	Sibling emigration	(not used)
Lambe_SyskonEmigrant2.txt	Sibling emigration2	(not used)

LINKAGE, DATA PROCESSING AND CONSTRUCTION OF ADDITIONAL VARIABLES

With the assistance of my data manager, Camilla Björk, I wrote programs in *SAS version 9.1.3 for UNIX* (Statistical Analysis System (SAS) Institute, 2006) to link the data from different registers, and to create new variables out of the existing data. Some of the operations performed were mundane formatting and data cleaning operations, such as removing extraneous characters from the variables and converting them into readable formats. The following description summarises the parts of the procedure that are of direct relevance to the project.

Retrieval of clinical data

The diagnoses that I defined as an episode of psychosis are listed in Table 4.11.

TABLE 4.11
ICD diagnoses retrieved from Hospital Discharge Register

Disorder	ICD–9	ICD–10
Schizophrenia	295, 295.A–G, W, X	F200–209
Schizoaffective disorder	295.H	F250–259
Bipolar affective disorder	296, 296.A, C–E, W, X	F300–319
Other non-affective psychosis	293, 294, 297, 298	F220–249, F289, 299

There were two problems relating to the classifications used in the ICD. First, the period of interest spanned the transition between ICD–9 and ICD–10. My approach was to use the ICD–10 definitions as the standard, and pick out the ICD–9 categories that most closely corresponded to them. However, it was not always obvious which ICD–9 categories to include under each diagnosis, particularly as ICD–9 retained the Kraepelinian concept of 'affective psychosis' (see page 5), which included severe unipolar depression as well as bipolar disorders. I therefore excluded the categories of 'major depression', but included 'manic disorder' and all varieties of 'bipolar affective disorder' (which includes depressive episodes within the context of a bipolar illness) under the 'bipolar affective disorder' category.

The second problem related to the distinction between illness episodes and lifetime diagnosis. My interest was in classifying individuals according to their 'lifetime' diagnosis. However, the data from the registers consisted of ICD codes for individual illness episodes. The process of converting a list of episode diagnoses into a lifetime diagnosis was not straightforward.

The ICD classification system is intended, and used, to characterise individual acute episodes. However, many of the categories in ICD allude to lifetime diagnoses: for example, 'bipolar disorder, current episode manic'. Despite including these lifetime diagnoses as part of the description of the acute episode, the ICD manual does not contain any guidance as to the diagnostic criteria for these lifetime diagnoses, or how they relate to the pattern of individual episodes.

I therefore devised the following procedure. I first listed all primary and secondary diagnoses for each individual, regardless of the order of the episodes, to give 16 permutations of the four diagnoses. I converted these to lifetime diagnoses using the algorithm in Table 4.12, which I believe reflects typical diagnostic practice, at least in the UK, in arriving at lifetime diagnoses. My guiding principle was to use a hierarchical diagnostic system, in which schizophrenia took precedence over all other diagnoses, followed by bipolar disorder and then schizoaffective disorder. Thus, a lifetime diagnosis of 'other psychosis' was only made in patients who had never received an episode diagnosis in any of the other three categories. I made one exception to the hierarchical rule: if schizophrenia and bipolar disorder

TABLE 4.12
Algorithm for converting permutations of illness episodes into lifetime diagnoses

Schizophrenia (1)	Schizoaffective (2)	Bipolar (3)	Other (4)	Lifetime diagnosis
0	0	0	0	None
0	0	0	1	Other
0	0	1	0	Bipolar
0	0	1	1	Bipolar
0	1	0	0	Schizoaffective
0	1	0	1	Schizoaffective
0	1	1	0	Bipolar
0	1	1	1	Bipolar
1	0	0	0	Schizophrenia
1	0	0	1	Schizophrenia
1	0	1	0	Schizoaffective
1	0	1	1	Schizoaffective
1	1	0	0	Schizophrenia
1	1	0	1	Schizophrenia
1	1	1	0	Schizoaffective
1	1	1	1	Schizoaffective

were both diagnosed in the same individual, I gave a lifetime diagnosis of schizoaffective disorder rather than schizophrenia. In some secondary analyses, the diagnostic procedure was changed; the details of these changes will be given in the descriptions of the individual analyses.

The age at onset was taken as the date of admission for the first index episode, regardless of whether the diagnosis at that episode matched the lifetime diagnosis.

Retrieval of school data

Where an individual appeared more than once in the School Register, indicating that the year had been repeated (less than 0.1% of all individuals, although over-represented (0.8%) in future schizophrenic patients), I used the data from the second year, for two reasons. First, the first year contained a much larger proportion of missing data. Second, since some children who repeated the year did so because of extenuating circumstances or unexpectedly poor grades in the first year, the repeated grades were probably a better indication of a student's cognitive ability than the original grades.

Rather than attempt to calculate grade-point average (GPA) from the individual subject scores, I used the GPA that was recorded in the database, since this took into account any decisions by the teacher to upgrade or downgrade pupils because of extenuating circumstances (such as cheating or illness), and also took into account information from optional subjects. The valid range for GPA was one to five. Where the GPA was given as zero (indicating that grades were missing), I generated an indicator variable that was used to exclude these individuals from the main analyses. I then calculated the mean and standard deviation (SD) of GPA for each sex, divided GPA by its SD and subtracted its mean to obtain standardised 'Z' scores, and then converted these into indicator variables (±1 SD, –1 to –2 SD, below –2 SD, etc.).

Parental data

Using the Multi-Generation Register, I linked in parental data on socio-economic group, education and country of origin. Educational level and socioeconomic group were listed for the 1980 and 1990 censuses for both parents. I took the highest value for either parent at either time-point and converted these to indicator variables.

I calculated parental ages at birth, and used this to generate binary variables for advanced paternal and maternal age. The cut-off for father's age at birth was initially set at 50 on the basis of previous research on schizophrenia in Sweden (Sipos et al., 2004), which had shown a marked increase in risk in men over 50. However, setting the threshold at 50 resulted in only 0.39% of the population exposed, with no exposed individuals in some diagnostic categories. I therefore reduced the cut-off to 45, giving 1.2% exposed, including at least two individuals in each diagnostic category. I then adjusted the cut-off for maternal age until approximately the same proportion of the population was classed as exposed, which occurred at a cut-off of 38 years.

Pregnancy and birth data

Birth measurements

Using Swedish reference data (Niklasson et al., 1991) and methods developed by Bergvall, Cnattingius and colleagues (2006), I standardised birthweight, length and head circumference for gestational age. The technique uses sex-specific distributions from a sample of Swedish infants born 1977–1981 (n=475,588). In the case of birthweight, where the data were positively skewed, I transformed the original skewed distributions for birthweight using the square root. I then generated categorical variables for high or low birthweight, length and head circumference, defined as greater than 2 SD above or below the sex-specific mean.

Apgar scores

For Apgar scores (a measure of the health of the newborn baby), I added a data check at the suggestion of Sven Cnattingius, one of my Swedish collaborators, who is an expert on the Medical Birth Register. The way that the data are entered makes it easy to confuse a score of 1 (indicating an unconscious, severely hypoxic neonate) and 10 (indicating a well-oxygenated neonate). Apgar scores almost invariably increase or stay the same at successive measurements. It is therefore almost certain that an apparent score change from 10 at 1 minute to 1 at 5 minutes is a data entry error. I therefore added an algorithm such that if the score at 1 minute was 10, but the score at 5 minutes was 1, the 5-minute score was reset to 10. I defined a categorical variable, hypoxia, as an Apgar score falling below 4 at any point.

Spring birth

I generated a 'spring birth' indicator variable for children born in January to April inclusive. I chose these months on the basis of previous research on an overlapping Swedish sample, suggesting that Jan–April birth was associated with later schizophrenia (Hultman et al., 1999).

Parity

Parity is the number of previous births to a foetus of ≥ 24 weeks' gestation. I generated an indicator variable for births to mothers whose parity was greater than 2.

Preterm delivery

I generated an indicator variable for preterm delivery if the number of completed weeks' gestation at birth was ≤ 36.

Calculation of entry and exit dates

For the subsequent survival analyses, I defined an entry and exit date for follow-up for every individual. Grades were awarded in June each year. In order to minimise the impact of any prodromal deterioration in functioning, I defined the entry date defined as 15 June in the year following the class 9 grade. I defined the exit date as the earliest of: first admission with the diagnosis being analysed; death; first emigration; or 31 December 2003.

Exclusion criteria

I imposed the following exclusion criteria:

- Born outside Sweden: these children were excluded to avoid confounding by migration status (see discussion).
- Either parent born outside Sweden: this was to avoid confounding by second-generation migration, as the schizophrenogenic effects of

migration appear to extend to at least the second generation (Cantor-Graae & Selten, 2005).

- Emigration at any time before the start of the observation period, even if the individual subsequently re-immigrated. These individuals were excluded because children who moved abroad during childhood may have experienced varying degrees of interruption to their schooling.
- Died or admitted with any index diagnosis prior to the start of the observation period.
- Missing data from both parents: information on at least one parent would be required to control for parental factors such as socioeconomic status.

ETHICAL APPROVAL

I obtained ethical approval from the respective ethics committees at Kings College London (Institute of Psychiatry) and the Karolinska Institutet, Stockholm.

CHAPTER FIVE

School performance and psychosis: unadjusted analyses

GENERAL

Aim

The aim of this chapter was to model the relationship between overall school performance at age 16, as measured by grade-point average (GPA), and time to psychosis, using a survival analysis. The chapter is divided into three sections. In the first section, I will describe the basic characteristics of the sample. In the next section, I will explore the crude relationship between school performance and psychosis, both overall and broken down by diagnosis. In the final section, I will explore the association between potential confounders and school performance, in preparation for the next chapter, where confounding and interaction will be considered in greater detail.

Software used

I performed all the analyses in this chapter using *Intercooled STATA 9.2 for Macintosh* (STATA, 2005), after using *StatTransfer 7* (StatTransfer, 2005) to convert the data file from SAS to STATA format.

Exclusions

I used the exclusion criteria defined on page 68. There were initially 907,011 pupils in the dataset. Of these, 181,596 individuals had at least one parent born outside Sweden, or missing data on both parents. In total 9404 had emigrated, 235 died, and 375 had been admitted with an index diagnosis prior to the start of follow-up; 715,401 remained.

Survival analysis

I set up a survival analysis, using the criteria defined on page 68. To allow easier interpretation, I re-scaled the *time* variable to years, and set the origin to date of birth, so that analysis time would be expressed in years of age. It should be noted that this re-scaling only affects how time is reported; the time used in the analysis (denoted $_t$ in *STATA*) remains as specified in on page 68, with time-zero defined, not as date of birth, but as 15 June in the year following the end of compulsory schooling.

I checked the ranges of all date variables, and dropped three observations as they contained impossible dates, leaving 715,398 subjects, with a total of 6,783,520 at risk. The earliest entry date was 14.83 years of age, and the last exit date was at 30.95 years of age.

The results of the regression analyses are presented using Poisson regression. I have also run unadjusted and fully adjusted analyses on all the outcomes using Cox regression for comparison, reported elsewhere (MacCabe et al., 2008; MacCabe et al., 2010). The results are almost identical using either technique.

Characteristics and coding of *medelbetyg*

Missing grades

Missing grades in individual school subjects

Including optional subjects, there were a total of 20 possible school subjects. Missing grades were found in individual subjects and for GPA – these did not necessarily coincide. In total 21,915 individuals (3.0% of the sample) had a missing grade in at least one subject. Common reasons for missing grades included non-attendance, being excused from a particular subject, being in residential care, or moving house at the time of the assessments.

Almost 90% (19,875) of those with at least one missing grade had sufficient data for a GPA to be calculated. About half (10,318) had only one missing grade, and the median number of missing grades for the remainder was 10. I therefore divided the number of missing grades into four categories: 0, 1, 2–10 and >10.

Table 5.1 shows the relationship between missing scores in individual subjects and GPA. Individuals with more missing scores had worse GPAs,

TABLE 5.1
The relationship between missing scores in individual subjects and grade-point average (GPA)

GPA Z-score	Number of missing grades (%)				
	0	1	2–10	>10	Total
Below –2	13,444	2,158	3,532	1,216	20,350
	(1.94)	(20.91)	(51.73)	(25.5)	(2.84)
–2 to –1	86,221	3,073	2,195	1,032	92,521
	(12.43)	(29.78)	(32.15)	(21.64)	(12.93)
–1 to +1 (ref)	487,313	4,314	978	468	493,073
	(70.27)	(41.81)	(14.32)	(9.81)	(68.92)
+1 to +2	96,981	714	89	35	97,819
	(13.98)	(6.92)	(1.3)	(0.73)	(13.67)
Over +2	8,701	59	7	5	8,772
	(1.25)	(0.57)	(0.1)	(0.1)	(1.23)
Missing	825	0	27	2,013	2,865
	(0.12)	(0)	(0.4)	(42.21)	(0.4)
Total	693,485	10,318	6,828	4,769	715,400
	(100)	(100)	(100)	(100)	(100)

and 42% of those with more than 10 missing scores had missing GPAs. All those with 18 or more missing grades had missing GPAs.

Missing grade-point average

In total 2,833 (0.3%) of the sample had a missing GPA. Of these 53% had 18 or more missing grades. Most of the remainder had no missing grades: the reasons for missing GPA were varied in these cases, but included children who moved between schools around the time of the assessment and other administrative reasons.

Since I had decided to use the GPA as recorded in the database, rather than attempt to calculate my own GPA, children with no GPA could not be included in the analyses for which GPA was the exposure, but I calculated the rate ratio for missing grades (reported below) before excluding them.

A histogram of *medelbetyg* (grade-point average) is shown in Figure 5.1.

Excluding the zeros, which indicated missing grades, GPA followed a normal distribution (the characteristic bell-shaped curve referred to in the title), with a mean of 3.25 and a standard deviation of 0.69. *Medelbetyg* was expressed to the nearest 0.1.

The distributions of both male and female scores showed a curious pattern: there seemed to be fewer children with scores that were exact integers, and there was also a suggestion that half-integers were also rarer

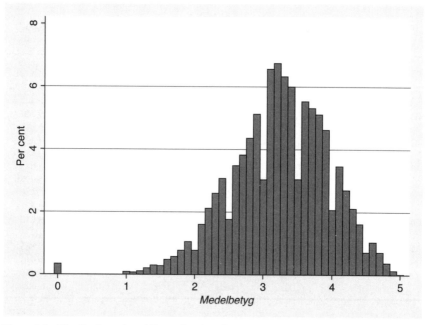

Figure 5.1 Distribution of *medelbetyg* (grade-point average)

than expected. Despite extensive investigation I have not been able to discover the reasons for this but I assume it is an artefact of the algorithm used by the Swedish authorities when rounding grade-point averages to the nearest 0.1 points. Since the points of rarity are evenly distributed and the scores still follow very close to a Gaussian distribution, I am confident that this should not bias the results.

I placed the cut-offs for calculating Z-score bands at 1.7/1.8, 2.4/2.5, 3.9/4.0 and 4.6/4.7. Figure 5.2 shows the distribution of *medelbetyg*, with the zeros omitted, showing the cut-offs used to calculate Z-score bands, with a normal distribution superimposed.

Figure 5.3 shows the same information in males (a) and females (b) separately.

The subjects were then categorised according to bands of differing performance. Individuals within one standard deviation of the mean (i.e. with a Z-score of ±1) were the reference category. The 'exposure' categories were: Z-score of ≤2, −2 to −1, +1 to +2, and ≥+2. The number of individuals in each category is shown in Table 5.2.

Females achieved considerably superior grades than males (Pearson chi-square $\chi^2=2.2\times104$, p<0.001).

Table 5.3 shows the distribution of Z-scores by diagnosis.

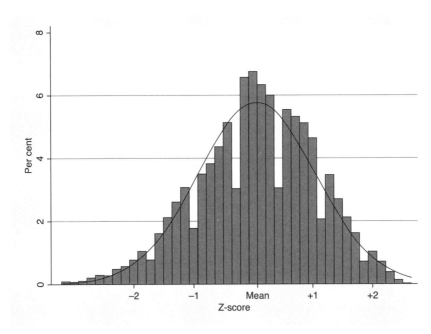

Figure 5.2 Z-score cut-off points for grade-point average (GPA) (zero scores excluded)

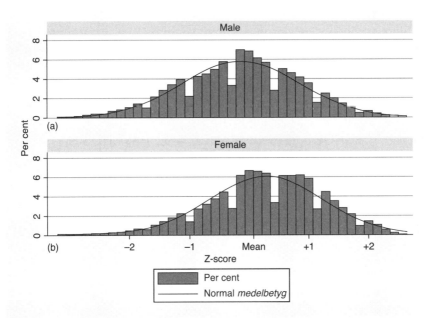

Figure 5.3 Histogram of grade-point average (GPA) (*medelbetyg*), by sex. (a) males; (b) females

TABLE 5.2
Distribution of grade-point average (GPA) Z-score band, by sex, and overall

GPA Z-score	Male n (%)	Female n (%)	Total n (%)
Below −2	14,412 (3.94)	5,938 (1.70)	20,350 (2.84)
−2 to −1	61,696 (16.85)	30,825 (8.82)	92,521 (12.93)
−1 to +1 (ref)	250,261 (68.37)	242,813 (69.50)	493,074 (68.92)
+1 to +2	35,757 (9.77)	62,062 (17.76)	97,819 (13.67)
Over +2	2,451 (0.67)	6,321 (1.81)	8,772 (1.23)
Missing	1,471 (0.40)	1,394 (0.40)	2,865 (0.40)
Total	366,048 (100.00)	349,353 (100.00)	715,401 (100.00)

Demographic details of the sample

Table 5.4 shows the demographic characteristics of the sample.

As expected, the clearest disparity in demographic data was that schizophrenia patients included a preponderance of males.

Figure 5.4 shows how family size was distributed in the population. It should be noted that family size for each individual was calculated using the number of full siblings in the sample, plus one. This is lower than the true number of full siblings, since some individuals had siblings who were outside the sample.

Since families of greater than 2 were relatively rare, I categorised both family size and birth order as 1, 2 or >2. Table 5.5 shows the relationship between family size, birth order and diagnosis. There was a greater proportion of only children in all four diagnostic groups.

CRUDE RELATIONSHIP BETWEEN OVERALL SCHOOL PERFORMANCE AND PSYCHOSIS

The analyses in this section are survival analyses (as defined on page 72), which take censoring into account, but are not adjusted for any confounders.

Combined psychoses

I began by combining all four disorders (schizophrenia, bipolar disorder, schizoaffective disorder and 'other psychoses') as the outcome: there were 1,780 cases over 6,783,520 person-years at risk, giving an overall incidence rate of 26 per 100,000 person-years for all psychoses. Mean age at onset was 21.83 years of age, with a standard deviation (SD) of 2.87, and a range of 16.73 to 29.71.

TABLE 5.3
Z-score category, by diagnosis

Z-score of GPA	No disorder (n=713,597)		Schizophrenia (n=493)		Schizoaffective disorder (n=95)		Bipolar disorder (n=280)		Other psychosis (n=936)	
	n	(%)	n	(%)	n	(%)	n	(%)	n	(%)
<–2	20,221	(2.8)	47	(9.6)	8	(8.5)	13	(4.7)	63	(6.7)
–2 to –1	92,150	(12.9)	104	(21.3)	26	(27.7)	38	(13.7)	207	(22.1)
–1 to +1	492,065	(69.0)	280	(57.3)	51	(54.3)	167	(60.1)	521	(55.7)
+1 to +2	97,603	(13.7)	48	(9.8)	7	(7.5)	48	(17.3)	114	(12.2)
>+2	8,750	(1.2)	0	(0.0)	0	(0.0)	10	(3.6)	12	(1.3)
Missing	2,833	(0.4)	10	(2.0)	2	(2.1)	2	(0.7)	19	
Repeated year	602		4		0		1		1	

The 'repeated year' category has no percentage because it is not an exclusive category. All subjects who repeated a year were included in the sample, and their latest grade was used. GPA, grade-point analysis.

TABLE 5.4
Demographic details of the sample

	No disorder (n=713,597)		Schizophrenia (n=493)		Schizoaffective disorder (n=95)		Bipolar disorder (n=280)		Other psychosis (n=936)	
	n	(%)	n	(%)	n	(%)	n	(%)	n	(%)
Male Sex	364,839	(51.0)	318	(64.5)	50	(52.6)	128	(45.7)	523	(55.9)
Parent's age at birth										
Father >45	8,497	(1.2)	14	(2.9)	2	(2.1)	7	(2.5)	17	(1.9)
Mother >38	9,719	(1.4)	12	(2.5)	1	(1.1)	5	(1.8)	15	(1.6)
Highest parental socioeconomic group										
SE/OC	60,024	(8.4)	69	(14.0)	10	(10.5)	1	(0.4)	106	(11.3)
WC higher	108,933	(15.3)	84	(17.0)	14	(14.7)	25	(8.9)	131	(14.0)
WC middle	92,678	(13.0)	56	(11.4)	12	(12.6)	41	(14.6)	107	(11.4)
WC lower	168,694	(23.6)	97	(19.7)	20	(21.1)	26	(9.3)	198	(21.1)
BC higher	153,708	(21.5)	109	(22.1)	20	(21.1)	74	(26.4)	235	(25.1)
BC lower	125,147	(17.5)	64	(13.0)	18	(19.0)	74	(26.4)	133	(14.2)
Missing	4,413	(0.6)	14	(2.84)	1	(1.1)	36	(12.9)	27	(2.9)
Highest parental education										
HE ≥3y	166,757	(23.4)	144	(29.2)	22	(23.2)	89	(31.8)	269	(28.7)
HE <3y	117,984	(16.5)	64	(13.0)	14	(14.7)	46	(16.4)	130	(13.9)
Hi schl 3 years	110,147	(15.4)	59	(12.0)	10	(10.5)	39	(13.9)	113	(12.1)
Hi schl 2 years	238,593	(33.4)	164	(33.3)	37	(39.0)	78	(28.0)	314	(33.5)
Compulsory only	76,644	(10.7)	59	(12.0)	12	(12.6)	25	(8.9)	100	(10.7)
Missing	3,472	(0.5)	3	(0.6)	0	(0)	3	(1.1)	11	(1.2)

GPA, grade-point average; SE/OC, self-employed/own company; WC, white collar; BC, blue collar; HE, higher education; Hi schl, high school.

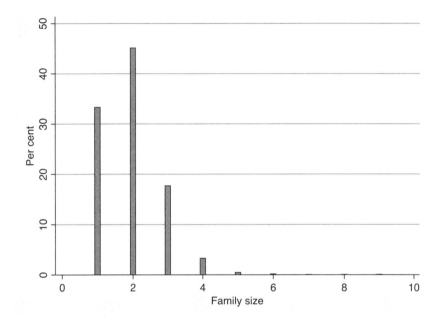

Figure 5.4   Histogram, showing the distribution of family size in the sample

Missing grades

Missing individual grades

The association between missing grades in individual subjects and all psychoses is shown in Figure 5.5. Compared with children with no missing grades, those with one missing grade had an incidence risk ratio (IRR) of 1.91 (95% CI 1.42 to 1.56; $\chi^2=18.8$, p<0.0001). The IRR for 2–10 missing grades was 3.81 (95% CI 2.95 to 4.91; $\chi^2=121.6$, p<0.0001), and for more than 10 missing grades was 5.28 (95% CI 4.06 tp 6.91; $\chi^2=184.5$, p<0.0001).

Missing grade point average

The IRR for all psychoses, comparing individuals with missing GPAs to individuals without missing grades was 5.30 (95% CI 3.76 to 7.48: $\chi^2=113.0$, p<0.0001).

Repeated grades

For individuals with repeated grades (regardless of their eventual grade), the equivalent IRR was 4.41 (95% CI 1.98 to 9.83; $\chi^2=15.8$, p=0.0001). It

TABLE 5.5
Family size and birth order, by diagnosis

Parameter	No disorder n (%)	Schizophrenia n (%)	Schizoaffective n (%)	Bipolar n (%)	Other psychosis n (%)	Total n (%)
Family size						
1	237,352 (33.26)	219 (44.79)	42 (44.68)	116 (41.73)	362 (39.43)	238,091 (33.28)
2	322,083 (45.13)	173 (35.38)	35 (37.23)	122 (43.88)	362 (39.43)	322,775 (45.12)
>2	154,186 (21.61)	97 (19.84)	17 (18.09)	40 (14.39)	194 (21.13)	154,534 (21.6)
Total	713,621 (100)	489 (100)	94 (100)	278 (100)	918 (100)	715,400 (100)
Birth order						
1	302,925 (42.45)	217 (44.38)	49 (52.13)	128 (46.04)	410 (44.66)	303,729 (42.46)
2	275,611 (38.62)	165 (33.74)	33 (35.11)	88 (31.65)	334 (36.38)	276,231 (38.61)
>2	135,085 (18.93)	107 (21.88)	12 (12.77)	62 (22.3)	174 (18.95)	135,440 (18.93)
Total	713,621 (100)	489 (100)	94 (100)	278 (100)	918 (100)	715,400 (100)

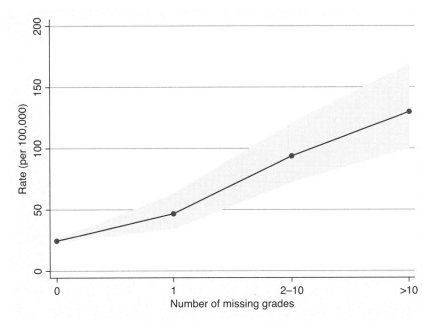

Figure 5.5   Rates of all psychoses by number of missing grades. Shaded area shows 95% confidence limits

should be noted that individuals with missing grades were excluded from further analyses, whereas those with repeated grades were included, using the later grades.

Overall rates by GPA category

The overall rates of psychosis in each category of GPA are shown in Figure 5.6.

Individuals with the poorest level of school performance had the highest incidence rates of psychosis (66.9 per 100,000 person-years), falling to 21.5 per 100,000 in the reference group (Table 5.6). The incidence rate of psychosis at higher levels of school performance was somewhat greater than in the reference category.

The crude incidence rate ratio (IRR) was 0.65 (95% confidence interval (CI) 0.61 to 0.70). In other words, for every increase of one standard deviation in GPA, risk for psychosis decreases by a factor of between 0.61 and 0.70.

However, this rate ratio assumes a linear relationship between Z-score band and risk for psychosis. This is problematic for two reasons. First, even if there were a linear relationship between Z-score *band* and risk for

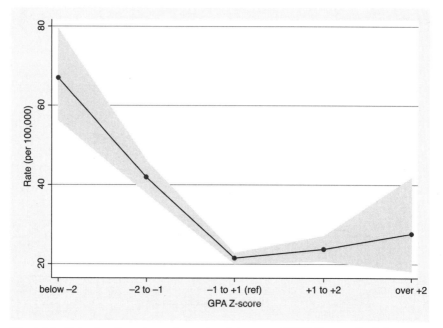

Figure 5.6 Rates for all psychoses, by grade-point average (GPA) Z-score. Shaded area
shows 95% confidence limits

TABLE 5.6
Rates of all psychoses by grade-point average (GPA) category

GPA Z-score	Cases	Person-years at risk (/100,000)	Rate (per 100,000 person-years)	95% confidence interval
Below –2	129	1.93	66.87	56.27 to 79.46
–2 to –1	371	8.86	41.86	37.81 to 46.35
–1 to +1 (ref)	1008	46.88	21.50	20.22 to 22.87
+1 to +2	216	9.13	23.67	20.71 to 27.04
Over +2	22	0.80	27.58	18.16 to 41.88

psychosis, this would not equate to a linear relationship between Z-score
itself and risk for psychosis, since the bands are of unequal widths (the '+1
to +2' and '–1 to –2' bands have a width of one standard deviation, the
reference band is twice as wide, whereas the lowest and highest bands have
no lower and upper limit respectively). Second, inspection of the rates in
Table 5.6 does not suggest such a linear relationship, and this was confirmed by a conducting a likelihood ratio (LR) test for departure from
linear trend, which strongly indicated a non-linear relationship (LR

TABLE 5.7
Poisson regression: hazard ratios for all psychoses at each grade-point average
(GPA) Z-score band

GPA Z-score	Hazard ratio	Standard error	z	p>z	95% confidence interval
Below −2	3.11	0.29	12.12	<0.001	2.59 to 3.73
−2 to −1	1.95	0.12	10.96	<0.001	1.73 to 2.19
−1 to +1 (ref)	1.00	–	–	–	– –
+1 to +2	1.10	0.08	1.27	0.206	0.95 to 1.27
Over +2	1.28	0.28	1.15	0.250	0.84 to 1.95

TABLE 5.8
Cox proportional hazards regression: hazard ratios for all psychoses at each grade-
point average (GPA) Z-score band

GPA Z-score	Hazard ratio	Standard error	z	p>z	95% confidence interval
Below −2	3.11	0.29	12.13	<0.001	2.59 to 3.73
−2 to −1	1.95	0.12	10.98	<0.001	1.73 to 2.19
−1 to +1 (ref)	1.00	–	–	–	– –
+1 to +2	1.09	0.08	1.2	0.229	0.94 to 1.27
Over +2	1.27	0.27	1.11	0.269	0.83 to 1.94

$\chi^2=69.04$ (3df), p<0.00001). We therefore need a more detailed analysis of the relationship between GPA and risk.

I therefore calculated individual rate ratios for each Z-score band, using the '+1 to –1' band as the reference category. Table 5.7 shows the results using Poisson regression. Individuals falling into the two lowest bands of performance were at significantly greater risk for psychosis than those in the reference category. Individuals with higher levels of performance had non-significantly elevated risks of psychosis.

For comparison, I performed the same analysis using Cox proportional hazards regression. A global test using Schoenfeld residuals showed no evidence that the proportional hazards assumption was violated ($\chi^2=3.40$ (4df), p=0.49) (Table 5.8).

Cox proportional hazards regression gave almost identical results to Poisson regression. Since Poisson regression is somewhat more flexible, and allows easier adjustment for age, I decided to use Poisson regression for the remainder of the analyses. As already noted, I repeated almost all these analyses using Cox regression, and obtained almost identical results. Indeed, the published version of my results used Cox regression (MacCabe et al., 2008, MacCabe et al., 2010).

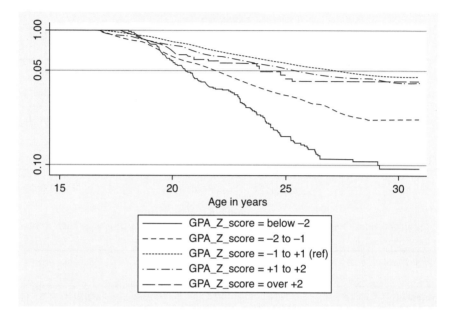

Figure 5.7 All psychoses: Kaplan–Meier plot. The y-axis is log-transformed to allow better discrimination between the curves. GPA, grade-point average

Graphical representations of rates of psychosis over time

The hazard ratio estimates above tell us about the overall rates of psychosis over the course of the follow-up period, but nothing about how these rates vary over time. The traditional method of showing rates over time is to plot the Kaplan–Meier survival function over time for all psychosis, at different levels of GPA score, as shown in Figure 5.7.

At the start of the follow-up period, all individuals are free of psychosis. The curve shows the probability of remaining free of psychosis to time t, taking censoring into account. Since psychosis is rare, even individuals with the lowest scores have an almost 100% probability of surviving psychosis-free until age 30, so a traditional Kaplan–Meier plot of these data would consist of five lines superimposed almost exactly on one another, running along the top of the figure. In Figure 5.7, I have therefore log-transformed the y-axis, so that the lines can be discriminated. However, this makes it difficult to interpret the relative slopes of the lines.

In my view, a more easily interpreted method of depicting changes in rates over time for rare outcomes is to plot the hazard function. Hazard refers to the instantaneous risk of developing psychosis at a given time,

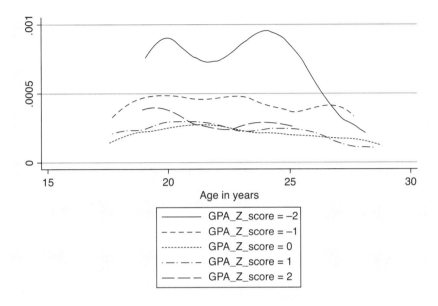

Figure 5.8 All psychoses: smoothed hazard estimates, by grade-point average (GPA) Z-score

conditional on having survived psychosis-free, until that point. Because hazard is an instantaneous measure, smoothing of the plot is needed to iron out day-to-day fluctuations in hazard.

Figure 5.8 shows the smoothed hazard functions for all psychoses, at different levels of GPA score. A hazard of 0.0005 corresponds to an incidence rate of 50 per 100,000 person-years.

Using this type of plot, the differing hazards at different levels of GPA score over time can be seen more clearly. The hazard among individuals in the lowest and second-lowest bands of GPA have consistently elevated hazard of psychosis throughout the age-range of the study, compared with the reference group. There is a suggestion that individuals in the lowest band have two peaks of incidence, at around age 20 and 24, but the more important result is that the hazard is greater than that for the other categories throughout this period.

Schizophrenia

There were 493 cases of schizophrenia, giving an overall incidence rate of 7 per 100,000 person-years, with a mean age of onset of 21.61 (SD 2.65, range 16.89–29.56), and a mean of 4.51 admissions (SD 5.45).

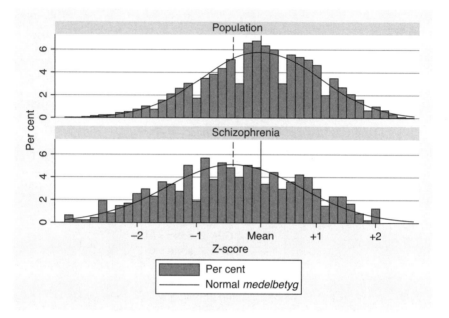

Figure 5.9 Distribution of grade-point average in schizophrenia and in the population. Dashed line indicates the mean for schizophrenia

TABLE 5.9
Rates of schizophrenia by grade-point average (GPA) category, showing hazard ratios and 95% confidence intervals, calculated using Poisson regression

GPA Z-score	Cases	Rate (per 100,000 person-years)	95% confidence interval	Hazard ratio	p>z	95% confidence interval
Below –2	47	24.36	18.30 to 32.43	4.08	<0.001	2.99 to 5.56
–2 to –1	104	11.74	9.68 to 14.22	1.97	<0.001	1.57 to 2.46
–1 to +1 (ref)	280	5.97	5.31 to 6.72	1.00	–	– –
+1 to +2	48	5.26	3.96 to 6.98	0.88	0.415	0.65 to 1.20
Over +2	0	0.00	– –	0.00	0.985	– to –

The IRR for missing grades was 5.85 (95% CI 3.13 to 10.95; χ^2=39.4, p<0.0001), and for repeated year was 10.75 (95% CI 4.02 to 28.75; χ^2=35.1, p<0.0001).

The distributions of grade-point average in schizophrenia compared with the population are shown in Figure 5.9. Patients with schizophrenia had the distribution of scores shifted to the left by 0.41 standard deviations.

The rates of schizophrenia in each GPA category are shown in Table 5.9, with hazard ratios and 95% confidence intervals calculated using Poisson

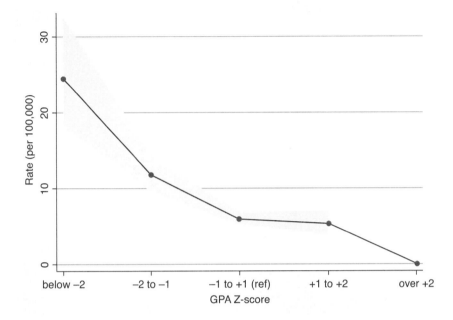

Figure 5.10 Rates of schizophrenia by grade-point average (GPA) Z-score. Shaded area shows 95% confidence limits

regression. Again, conducting the same analysis using Cox proportional hazards regression gave identical results (no hazard ratios or confidence intervals differed by more than 0.01 between models; results not presented). The results are presented graphically in Figure 5.10.

There is a clear reduction in risk of schizophrenia with every increase in school performance. It is notable that there were no cases of schizophrenia in the highest band.

Figure 5.11 shows a simple scatterplot of age at onset and GPA in cases of schizophrenia. There is no evidence of any relationship between GPA and age at onset (Pearson's r=0.0036, p=0.938). Figure 5.12 shows the smoothed hazard estimates for schizophrenia, by GPA level, showing that the association between GPA and schizophrenia is consistent at all ages of onset. Note that GPA score above +2 is not shown, as there are no cases of schizophrenia in that category.

Schizoaffective disorder

There were 94 cases of schizoaffective disorder, with an overall incidence rate of 1 per 100,000 person-years and a mean age at onset of 21.48 (SD 2.88, range 17.06–28.97). The mean number of admissions was 4.90 (SD 4.75).

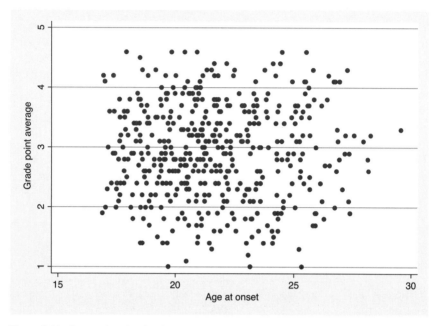

Figure 5.11 Scatterplot showing how grade-point average (*medelbetyg*) varies with age at onset in schizophrenia

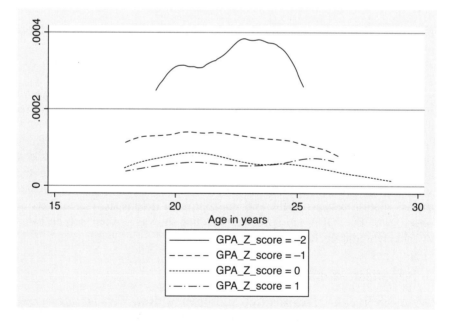

Figure 5.12 Schizophrenia: hazard estimates by grade-point average (GPA) Z-score

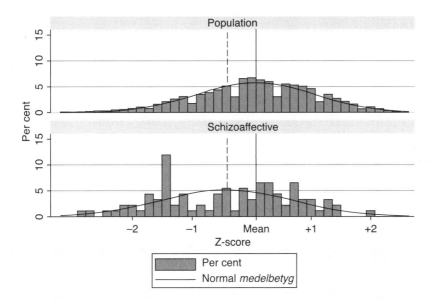

Figure 5.13 Distribution of grade-point average in schizoaffective disorder and in the population. The means and standard deviations are shown for the population. Dashed line indicates the mean for schizoaffective disorder

The IRR for missing grades was 6.09 (95% CI 1.50 to 24.74; χ^2=8.34, p=0.004). There were no cases of schizoaffective disorder in pupils who had repeated years.

Figure 5.13 shows the distribution of GPA in the schizoaffective patients and in the population. The pattern is similar to that for schizophrenia, with the entire distribution shifted to the left by 0.43 standard deviations.

The rates of schizoaffective disorder in each GPA category are shown in Table 5.10 and Figure 5.14.

The pattern of findings is very similar to that of schizophrenia, with a reduction in risk for disorder with every consecutive increase in GPA band. However, the hazard estimates are less constant over time than for schizophrenia; in particular, individuals with GPA Z-score of less than –2 who develop schizoaffective disorder, tend to have a somewhat earlier onset than individuals with higher scores (Figure 5.15), with no onsets after age 23.6 (mean age of onset in 'below –2' category=20.39, SD 1.63, range 18.38–23.63).

While cases in the lowest *medelbetyg* category do have earlier onsets, there is little overall relationship between age at onset and GPA in schizoaffective disorder (Pearson's r=0.012, p=0.907). This can be seen in the

TABLE 5.10
Rates of schizoaffective disorder by grade-point average (GPA) category, showing
hazard ratios and 95% confidence intervals, calculated using Poisson regression

GPA Z-score	Cases	Rate (per 100,000 person-years)	95% confidence interval	Hazard ratio	p>z	95% confidence interval
Below –2	8	4.15	2.07 to 8.29	3.81	<0.001	1.81 to 8.03
–2 to –1	26	2.93	2.00 to 4.31	2.70	<0.001	1.68 to 4.33
–1 to +1 (ref)	51	1.09	0.83 to 1.43	1.00	–	– –
+1 to +2	7	0.77	0.37 to 1.61	0.71	0.386	0.32 to 1.55
Over +2	0	0.00	– –	0.00	0.982	– to –

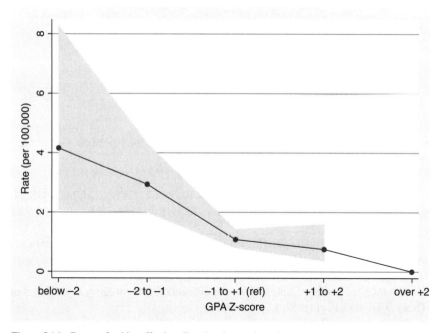

Figure 5.14   Rates of schizoaffective disorder, by grade-point average (GPA) Z-score.
Shaded area shows 95% confidence limits

scatterplot at age of onset against GPA in patients with schizoaffective
disorder (Figure 5.16). The horizontal line shows the threshold for the
'below –2' category, so cases below this line are responsible for the 'below
–2' line in Figure 5.15.

As with schizophrenia, it should be noted that there is no 'above +2'
category, as no individuals in that category developed schizoaffective
disorder.

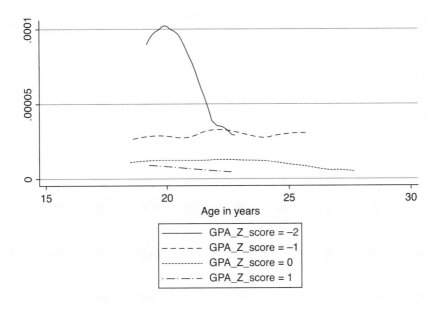

Figure 5.15 Schizoaffective disorder: smoothed hazard estimates by grade-point average (GPA) Z-score

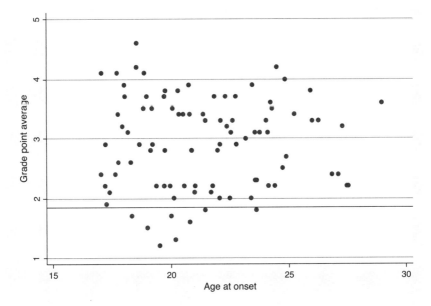

Figure 5.16 Scatterplot showing how grade-point average (*medelbetyg*) varies with age at onset in schizoaffective disorder. Cases below the line are in the lowest *medelbetyg* category and tend to have a younger age at onset

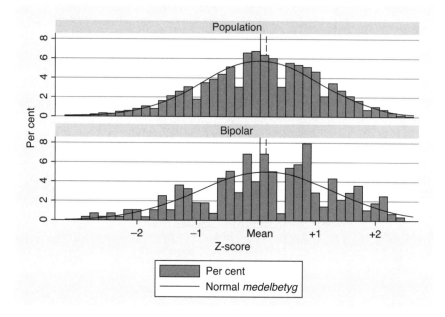

Figure 5.17 Distribution of grade-point average in bipolar disorder and in the population. The means and standard deviations are shown for the population. Dashed line indicates the mean for bipolar disorder

Bipolar disorder

There were 278 cases of bipolar disorder, with a mean age of onset of 20.79 years (SD 2.73, range 16.73–29.14). The mean number of admissions was 2.50 (SD 2.65). The incidence rate was 4 per 100,000. Unlike schizophrenia or schizoaffective disorder, individuals who missed or repeated a year did not have significantly elevated rates of bipolar disorder (hazard ratio (HR) for missing=2.03 (95% CI 0.51 to 8.16; χ^2=1.04, p=0.31); HR for repeated year=4.71 (95% CI=0.66 to 33.51; χ^2=2.9, p=0.09)).

Figure 5.17 shows the rates distribution of GPA in bipolar disorder compared with the population. The distribution of scores is shifted very slightly upwards (by 0.09 standard deviations), and there is an excess of bipolar subjects in the upper and lower tails of the distribution.

Table 5.11 and Figure 5.18 show the rates of bipolar disorder by GPA Z-score category. Individuals in the lowest category have moderately increased risk for bipolar disorder, although the risk for bipolar is small compared with that for schizophrenia or schizoaffective disorder. Furthermore, in contrast to the other disorders, risks for bipolar disorder are significantly greater in the highest and second-highest category of school

TABLE 5.11
Rates of bipolar disorder by grade-point average (GPA) category, showing hazard ratios and 95% confidence intervals, calculated using Poisson regression

GPA Z-score	Cases	Rate (per 100,000 person-years)	95% confidence interval	Hazard ratio	p>z	95% confidence interval
Below −2	13	6.74	3.91 to 11.61	1.89	0.027	1.08 to 3.33
−2 to −1	38	4.29	3.12 to 5.89	1.20	0.302	0.85 to 1.71
−1 to +1 (ref)	167	3.56	3.06 to 4.15	1.00	–	– –
+1 to +2	48	5.26	3.96 to 6.98	1.48	0.017	1.07 to 2.04
Over +2	10	12.53	6.74 to 23.30	3.52	<0.001	1.86 to 6.66

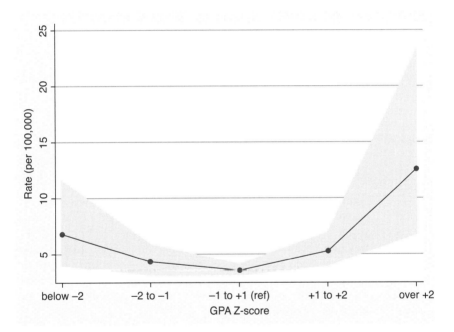

Figure 5.18 Rates of bipolar disorder, by grade-point average (GPA) Z-score. Shaded area shows 95% confidence limits

performance. In the highest (>+2) category, this difference is particularly marked, with a hazard ratio of 3.5, as compared with hazard ratios of zero for both schizophrenia and schizoaffective disorder.

Like for the other diagnoses, I repeated these analyses using Cox regression, and obtained almost identical results (not shown).

Figure 5.19 shows the hazard for bipolar disorder over time. It is notable that individuals who were in the highest band tended to have particularly early onsets (mean age of onset in 'above +2' 19.22, SD 1.24, range

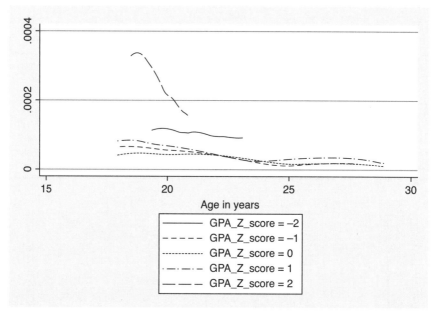

Figure 5.19 Bipolar disorder: smoothed hazard estimates by grade-point average (GPA) Z-score

17.72–21.60). However, as with the lowest category in schizoaffective disorder, it is important to note that this band contained a relatively small number of individuals compared with the other bands. Figure 5.20 shows a scatterplot of age at onset against GPA in patients with bipolar disorder. The horizontal line shows the threshold for the 'above +2' category, so cases above this line are responsible for the 'over +2' line in Figure 5.19. Although there is little overall relationship between age at onset and GPA (Pearson's r=−0.035, p=0.563), it is clear from Figure 5.20 that those in the 'above +2' category have earlier onsets.

It is possible that undetected prodromal symptoms of hypomania, could improve the ability of the students to study and perform well in examinations, and that this could explain the earlier onsets in those with excellent performance. As I have explained, I had attempted to obviate any reverse causation of this kind by excluding individuals first admitted to hospital within 1 year of their class 9 exams. To assess the effects of reverse causality, I doubled this period of exclusion to 2 years and observed very little change in the findings (HR for '>+2SD'=3.29 (95% CI 1.62 to 6.72); HR for '−<2SD' = 2.08 (95% CI 1.15 to 3.75)). Excluding a third year, however, resulted in the exclusion of 95 (one-third) of the cases of bipolar disorder and a loss of statistical significance (HR for '>+2SD'=1.97 (95% CI 0.73 to 5.34); HR for '−<2SD'=2.28 (95% CI 1.23 to 4.23)).

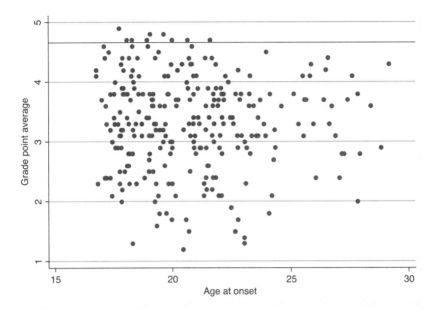

Figure 5.20 Scatterplot showing how grade-point average (*medelbetyg*) varies with age at onset in bipolar disorder. Cases above the line are in the highest *medelbetyg* category and tend to have a younger age at onset

CHAPTER SIX

Confounding and interaction: finding the model that best describes the data

DEFINITION OF CONFOUNDING AND EFFECT MODIFICATION

A confounder is a factor that can either cause or prevent the outcome of interest, is not on the causal pathway, but is also statistically associated with the exposure of interest (Last, 2001). Failure to detect and control for confounders can lead to, or accentuate, a statistical association between an exposure and an outcome. A confounder may exaggerate or mask a true association. For example, in this study, I have demonstrated a statistical association between the school performance and psychosis, but that association may not be causal. If the real causal association is between, say, socioeconomic group and psychosis, and if socioeconomic group is statistically associated with school performance, then school performance will show a statistical association with psychosis, and thus masquerade as a cause. In this situation, socioeconomic group would be a confounder.

Some confounders are measured, others are not. Unmeasured confounding cannot be detected or prevented in an observational study such as this. Measured confounders, however, can be identified and dealt with using multivariable regression techniques. Some measured confounders are completely and accurately measured: gender, for example. The measurement of some confounders, such as socioeconomic conditions, may be inaccurate, incomplete or imprecise, resulting in some residual confounding despite attempts to statistically adjust for confounding.

Effect modification (synonymous with interaction) describes a situation in which the relationship between the exposure and outcome differs, depending on the level of a third variable. For example, if the association between school performance and risk for psychosis diminishes as the subjects age, then age is acting as an effect modifier, or there is an interaction between school performance and age on risk for psychosis.

MODELLING APPROACH

It is common in published literature to simply include all variables that could theoretically be confounding the association in a regression equation. This has the desired effect of producing estimates that are minimally confounded by the variables in question, but there are two problems with this technique. First, the inclusion in a model of variables that are not actually confounding the association tends to inflate the standard errors of all estimates, and thus produce unnecessarily imprecise estimates. Second, there is no exploration of the effects of individual variables, including effect modification (interaction).

I have therefore employed a forward-fitting approach to the analysis of confounders. First, I will identify which of the variables that I have measured are likely to be confounders or effect modifiers, using my knowledge of the field and assisted by the data. In particular, I will only consider variables as potential confounders if they are statistically associated with school performance and psychosis, since both these conditions must be met for the variable to be confounding the association.

Since interactions increase the number of terms in a model in a multiplicative way, there is little to be gained from specifying every possible interaction, since the resulting model becomes rapidly unwieldy and uninterpretable, particularly in this case, where the exposure itself contributes four terms to the model, each of which would have an interaction term with every level of every interacting variable. I will therefore only test for interactions where I have specific *a priori* hypotheses that interaction is occurring. This is the case for age and sex only.

In the case of age, the hypothesis to be tested is that some of the apparent association between school performance and psychosis is due to prodromal effects. In other words, individuals perform poorly (or well) at school because they have an undetected prodromal illness. If this were the case, one would expect patients with a younger age at onset to have a stronger association between school performance and psychosis that those with an older age at onset. This would manifest as an interaction between school performance and age at onset.

In the case of sex, the great majority of previous studies in this area have used males only – it is therefore important to confirm that the same associations exist in females, i.e. that there is no interaction between school performance and sex.

I built up a regression model adding confounders and/or effect modifiers one by one, starting with the most likely or important. As different variables and interaction terms were added, I assessed the effect of these changes to the model on the associations between school performance and risk of psychosis. When the addition of further variables did not make a clear difference to the association between school performance and psychosis, I arrived at a model that describes the data as parsimoniously as possible, but contains no unnecessary parameters. Using this type of approach, the process of adding confounders along the way is informative, and for that reason I have shown the entire process of model fitting in an appendix. In the main text I have presented the final model.

ASSOCIATIONS OF POTENTIAL CONFOUNDERS WITH SCHOOL PERFORMANCE

As explained on page 98, only variables that are associated with the exposure of interest should be considered as potential confounders. I therefore tested the association between the potential confounders and/or effect modifiers and grade-point average (GPA).

To allow clearer presentation, I divided the potential confounders into characteristics of the individual, and those operating at the family level. Figure 6.1 shows how the mean GPA for the entire sample varies according to the individual-level confounders.

The horizontal line shows the overall mean GPA, and the points show the mean GPA for each level of the confounders. It is particularly notable that females score much more highly than males. Children born in late winter had marginally better scores than those born during the rest of the year. This is probably an artefact of the Swedish education system, where the cut-off for assignment to each year group is 1 January. Children born earlier in the year are thus the oldest in their class, and thus more developmentally mature than their classmates. Finally, first-born children perform better than second-born ones, who perform better than later-born children. This may in part be related to the tendency of larger families to have poorer scores (see Figure 6.2). Age band refers to age at exit from the study, and was divided into <20, 20–25 and >25. Not surprisingly, age band had no association with GPA; if it did, this would suggest that mean GPA scores were changing over time, and this would indicate an error in the peer-referencing of scores within the Swedish education system (see page 49).

Figure 6.2 shows how family-related variables are related to GPA. As expected, there is a strong correlation between both parental education and

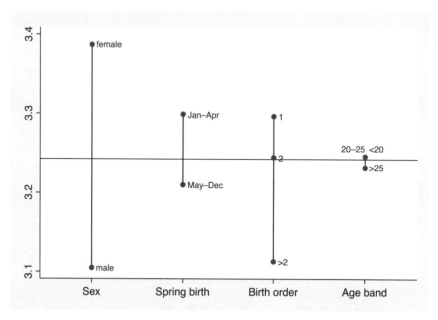

Figure 6.1   Means of *medelbetyg* (grade-point average), by individual-level confounders

socioeconomic group and school performance. The only exception is that the 'highest' socioeconomic group (group 6) according to the classification does not have the highest scores. This is a heterogeneous group that includes owners of large and successful companies along with owners of very small businesses, self-employed freelance workers and farmers. It is therefore not clear how it might relate to the other five categories of employees, which have a clear hierarchy. It will be important to bear this in mind when controlling for confounding, as it will probably not be correct to treat this as an ordered categorical variable, unless category 6 is treated as missing. Parental age had little association with grades. 'Only' children (who may nevertheless have had siblings outside the sample) appeared to have lower scores than children with siblings.

Low, but not high birthweight, birth length and head circumference were associated with lower scores, as were preterm delivery and neonatal hypoxia (Figure 6.3).

Relationship between grade-point average and number of admissions

Figure 6.4 shows the relationship between GPA and number of admissions in each diagnostic group. There is no evidence that subjects with low grades have more admissions.

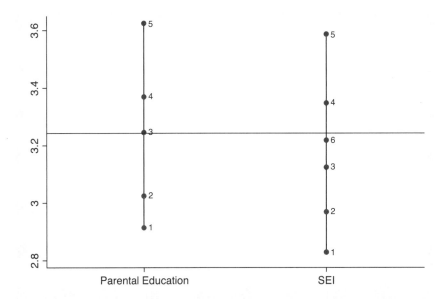

Figure 6.2   Means of *medelbetyg* (grade-point average), by family-level confounders. Parental_edu, parental education level: (1) compulsory school only (9 years), (2) upper secondary school (2 years), (3) upper secondary school (3 years), (4) higher education (<3 years), and (5) higher education (≥3 years); Sei_cat, socioeconomic status: (1) blue collar, unskilled, (2) blue collar, skilled (3) white collar (lower), (4) white collar (middle), (5) white collar (higher), (6) company owner/self-employed

SCHIZOPHRENIA: CONFOUNDING AND INTERACTION

Association of possible confounders or effect modifiers with schizophrenia risk

It was clear from the analyses presented in the previous chapter that there was a strong statistical association between school performance and schizophrenia. The purpose of this chapter was to identify variables that might be confounding this association. To be a confounder, a variable must be associated with the exposure, and also a risk factor for the outcome of interest (see page 97). I therefore began by testing for crude associations between potential confounders and risk for schizophrenia, before deciding which variables to add to my multivariable regression model.

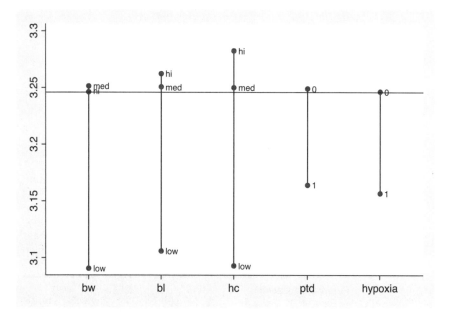

Figure 6.3 Means of medelbetyg (grade-point average), by birth characteristics. Bw, birthweight; bl, birth length; hc, head circumference; low, at least 2 SD below population mean; hi, at least 2 SD above population mean; ptd, preterm delivery (<36 completed weeks of gestation); hypoxia, any Apgar score <4

Age

Table 6.1 shows the rate of schizophrenia in three different age bands. There is a tendency for the rate of psychosis to be lower in people who remain well until age 26 or over. However, this was non-significant (rate ratio (RR) for 1 year increase in age=0.997(95% CI 0.988 to 1.005; χ^2=0.53, p=0.46)).

Sex

Males had nearly double the risk of schizophrenia compared to females (Table 6.2) (IRR=1.85 (95% CI 1.53 to 2.23) χ^2=42.6, p<0.0001).

Socioeconomic group

Socioeconomic group had a strong relationship to schizophrenia, with subjects in lower groups having higher rates of schizophrenia. Table 6.3

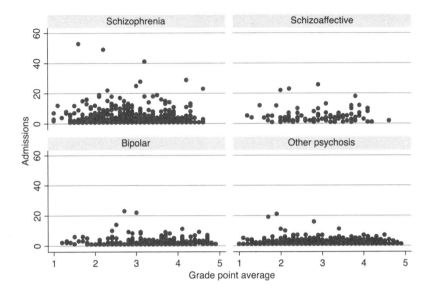

Figure 6.4   Grade-point average and number of admissions, by diagnostic group

shows the rates of schizophrenia by socioeconomic group. There was an RR of 0.89 (95% CI 0.84 to 0.94; χ^2=16.0, p=0.0001) for each increase in socioeconomic group.

Family size

The rate of schizophrenia was higher in sibships with only one individual and in those with more than two (Table 6.4). There was a tendency for rates to increase with increasing family size, but the numbers were too small to be meaningful for larger families. For subsequent analyses, I used a dichotomous variable indicating 2 or more in the sibship (RR for schizophrenia=1.4 (95% CI 1.17 to 1.68; χ^2=14.0, p=0.0002)).

Parental education level

Parental education level had a U-shaped relationship with risk for schizophrenia; individuals with highly educated and poorly educated parents had the higher rates of schizophrenia than those with intermediate levels of education (Table 6.5). However, there was no evidence of any trend for rates of schizophrenia to increase or decrease with parental education (RR

TABLE 6.1
Rates of schizophrenia, by age

Age band	n	Rate (/100,000)	95% confidence interval
<20	153	7.1	6.1 to 8.4
20–25	271	8.5	7.6 to 9.6
>25	65	4.5	3.5 to 5.7

TABLE 6.2
Rates of schizophrenia, by sex

Sex	n	Rate (/100,000)	95% confidence interval
Male	323	9.3	8.3 to 10.4
Female	166	5.0	4.3 to 5.9

TABLE 6.3
Rates of schizophrenia by socioeconomic group: note that 1
denotes the lowest socioeconomic group, 6 the highest

Socioeconomic group	n	Rate (/100,000)	95% confidence interval
1	69	12.1	9.5 to 15.3
2	82	8.0	6.4 to 9.9
3	55	6.3	4.8 to 8.2
4	97	6.1	5.1 to 7.4
5	108	7.4	6.1 to 9.0
6	64	5.3	4.1 to 6.8

TABLE 6.4
Rates of schizophrenia, by number in sibship

Number in sibship	n	Rate (/100,000)	95% confidence interval
1	219	8.81	7.72 to 10.06
2	173	5.90	5.08 to 6.85
3	72	6.46	5.12 to 8.13
4	16	7.76	4.76 to 12.67
5	6	17.33	7.79 to 38.58
6	1	12.92	1.82 to 91.74
7	2	98.93	24.74 to 395.55
8	0	0.00	– –
9	0	0.00	– –

TABLE 6.5
Rates of schizophrenia, by parents' highest education level

Parental education level	n	Rate (/100,000)	95% confidence interval
1	59	7.64	5.92 to 9.86
2	163	7.15	6.13 to 8.34
3	58	5.52	4.27 to 7.14
4	63	5.74	4.48 to 7.34
5	143	9.24	7.84 to 10.88

TABLE 6.6
Rates of schizophrenia, by pregnancy outcomes

Pregnancy/birth outcome	n	Rate (/100,000)	95% confidence interval
Birthweight			
High	8	5.33	2.67 to 10.67
Medium	463	7.24	6.61 to 7.93
Low	18	7.50	4.72 to 11.90
Birth length			
High	11	6.53	3.61 to 11.78
Medium	466	7.31	6.67 to 8.00
Low	12	5.02	2.86 to 8.85
Head circumference			
High	8	5.85	2.92 to 11.69
Medium	461	7.16	6.53 to 7.85
Low	20	9.51	6.14 to 14.74
Gestational age			
≥36	467	7.13	6.51 to 7.81
<36	22	9.32	6.14 to 14.16
Apgar scores			
All ≥4	484	7.19	6.57 to 7.86
Any <4	5	10.25	4.26 to 24.62

estimate for one unit increase in parental education level=1.05 (95% CI 0.98 to 1.12; χ^2=1.9, p=0.17)).

Pregnancy and birth characteristics

None of the adverse pregnancy outcomes analysed had any statistically significant associations with schizophrenia (Table 6.6).

Other variables

Paternal age over 45 was significantly associated with risk for schizophrenia (RR=2.43 (95% CI 1.43 to 4.13; χ^2=11.4, p=0.0007)), but since this was not related to school performance, it could not have been acting as a confounder.

Spring birth, birth order and maternal age >38 had no statistically significant associations with schizophrenia.

Schizophrenia – modelling strategy

From the previous analyses, it seemed likely that sex and socioeconomic group may be confounding the association between school performance and schizophrenia, since both these variables were strongly associated with both school performance and risk for schizophrenia. Family size seemed also to be a possible confounder. Parental education was also strongly associated with school performance, although its relationship to schizophrenia was U-shaped. I wanted to explore further the relationship between GPA, parental education and risk for schizophrenia.

With regard to interactions, I hypothesised that early-onset schizophrenia might be more strongly associated with poor school performance than later-onset schizophrenia, because of prodromal effects. I also wished to stratify by gender: not because I strongly suspected that any interaction was present, but because most previous studies on pre-morbid cognitive performance and schizophrenia have used only males, so I wanted to assess whether any association was present separately in females as well as males.

Schizophrenia – results

Please see the appendix for details of the modelling process. Overall, the association between poor school performance and schizophrenia was not explained by confounding. The association between school performance and schizophrenia was confounded to some extent by sex, socioeconomic group and family size, although the association remained very strong even after adjusting for these confounders. The association was not confounded by parental education. There was no evidence that subjects with an earlier age of onset had a worse school performance than those with a later age of onset. There was no evidence that the association between school performance and schizophrenia differed between males and females, or according to parental education. The model with the most parsimonious fit is shown in Table 6.7.

TABLE 6.7
Hazard ratios for schizophrenia, adjusted for sex, socioeconomic
group and family size

Parameter	Hazard ratio	p>z	95% confidence interval
GPA Z-score			
−2	3.54	<0.001	2.56 to 4.89
−2 to −1	1.71	<0.001	1.35 to 2.17
−1 to +1 (ref)	1.00	–	– –
+1 to +2	0.95	0.755	0.70 to 1.30
Over +2	0.00	0.975	– –
Female	0.58	<0.001	0.47 to 0.70
Socioeconomic group (SEG)			
SEG 1	1.51	0.012	1.09 to 2.09
SEG 2	1.15	0.354	0.85 to 1.56
SEG 3	0.95	0.765	0.68 to 1.33
SEG 5	1.34	0.039	1.01 to 1.78
SEG 6	0.83	0.261	0.60 to 1.15
Family size>1	1.24	0.021	1.03 to 1.49

GPA, grade-point average.

SCHIZOAFFECTIVE DISORDER: CONFOUNDING AND INTERACTION

Association of possible confounders with schizoaffective disorder risk

Birth order

There was a barely significant trend (RR=0.76 (95% CI 0.58 to 1.00; χ^2 for trend=3.88, p=0.049)) for first-born children to have higher rates of schizoaffective disorder than second-born children, and for second-born children to have higher rates than later-born children (Table 6.8).

Preterm delivery

There was a significant association between preterm delivery and schizo-affective disorder ((RR=2.32 (95% CI 1.03 to 4.82; χ^2=4.41, p=0.036)) (Table 6.9).

Other variables

There was no statistically significant association of sex, spring birth, family size, socioeconomic group, parental education, advanced paternal or maternal age with risk for schizoaffective disorder.

TABLE 6.8
Rates of schizoaffective disorder, by birth order

Birth order	n	Rate (/100,000)	95% confidence interval
1	49	1.69	1.27 to 2.23
2	33	1.26	0.90 to 1.78
>2	12	0.95	0.54 to 1.67

TABLE 6.9
Rates of schizoaffective disorder, by preterm delivery

Gestational age at birth	n	Rate (/100,000)	95% confidence interval
≥36 weeks (ref)	87	1.33	1.08 to 1.64
<36 weeks (preterm)	7	2.97	1.41 to 6.22

Schizoaffective disorder – modelling strategy

Preterm delivery was associated with poor performance in school and also with increased risk for schizoaffective disorder, so this could be acting as a confounder.

Earlier-born children had higher rates of schizoaffective disorder than later-born children. However, earlier-born children did better at school that later-born children, so there was the possibility of negative confounding (i.e. a true association being masked, as opposed to exaggerated, by the confounder).

In addition to controlling for the above confounders, I also stratified on sex and age, for the reasons given on page 106.

Schizoaffective disorder – results

Please see the appendix for details of the modelling process. Like schizophrenia, there was very little confounding overall. The data were best described by a model including preterm delivery and birth order, shown in Table 6.10. There was evidence of a modest degree of confounding by preterm delivery, and some negative confounding by birth order. There was no evidence that subjects with an earlier age at onset had a worse school performance than those with a later age of onset, or that the association between school performance and schizophrenia differed substantially between males and females.

TABLE 6.10
Hazard ratios for schizoaffective disorder, adjusted for preterm
delivery and birth order

Parameter	Hazard ratio	p>z	95% confidence interval
GPA Z-score			
Below −2	3.99	0.000	1.89 to 8.43
−2 to −1	2.77	0.000	1.73 to 4.45
−1 to +1 (ref)	1.00	–	– –
+1 to +2	0.69	0.354	0.31 to 1.52
Over +2	0.00	0.982	– –
Preterm delivery	1.82	0.158	0.79 to 4.16
Birth order			
Second born	0.73	0.159	0.46 to 1.13
Third born or greater	0.50	0.033	0.27 to 0.94

GPA, grade-point average.

BIPOLAR DISORDER: CONFOUNDING AND INTERACTION

Association of possible confounders with bipolar disorder risk

Age

There was a strong association between risk for bipolar disorder and age, with higher rates in lower age groups (Table 6.11). The risk ratio for a 1-year increase in age was 0.97 (95% CI 0.95 to 0.98; χ^2 for trend=37.6, p<0.0001).

Parental education

There was a linear association between parental education level and risk for bipolar disorder, whereby children with better educated parents were at increased risk of bipolar (Table 6.12). The risk ratio for one increase in parental education level was 1.16 (95% CI 1.07 to 1.27; χ^2 for trend=11.8, p=0.0006).

Paternal age

Paternal age over 45 at birth was associated with risk for bipolar disorder (RR=2.13 (95% CI 1.00 to 4.50; χ^2=4.0, p=0.044)) (Table 6.13).

TABLE 6.11
Rates of bipolar disorder, by age at onset

Age band	n	Rate (/100,000)	95% confidence interval
<20	132	6.15	5.19 to 7.30
20–25	119	3.74	3.12 to 4.47
>25	27	1.86	1.27 to 2.71

TABLE 6.12
Rates of bipolar disorder, by highest parental education level

Parental education level	n	Rate (/100,000)	95% confidence interval
1	25	3.24	2.19 to 4.79
2	78	3.42	2.74 to 4.27
3	39	3.71	2.71 to 5.08
4	45	4.10	3.06 to 5.49
5	88	5.68	4.61 to 7.00

TABLE 6.13
Rates of bipolar disorder, by paternal age at birth

Paternal age at birth	n	Rate (/100,000)	95% confidence interval
≥45	271	4.04	3.59 to 4.55
>45	7	8.59	4.10 to 18.02

Pregnancy and birth characteristics

Small head circumference (RR for a 2 SD increase in head circumference=0.57 (95% CI 0.034 to 0.69); χ^2 for trend=4.5, p=0.034) and preterm delivery (RR=2.04 (95% CI 1.28 to 3.24; χ^2=9.32, p=0.002)) were statistically associated with increased risk for bipolar disorder (Table 6.14). This was an unexpected finding, since a recent meta-analysis concluded that bipolar disorder was probably not associated with obstetric complications (Scott et al., 2006).

Other variables

There was no statistically significant association of sex, socioeconomic group, spring birth, birth order, family size or advanced maternal age and risk for bipolar disorder.

TABLE 6.14
Rates of bipolar disorder, by pregnancy and birth characteristics

Pregnancy/birth outcome	n	Rate (/100,000)	95% confidence interval
Head circumference			
High	4	2.92	1.10 to 7.79
Medium	259	4.02	3.56 to 4.55
Low	15	7.13	4.30 to 11.83
Gestational age			
≥36	259	3.96	3.50 to 4.47
<36	19	8.05	5.13 to 12.62

Bipolar disorder – modelling strategy

The incidence rate of bipolar was clearly much higher in younger patients, so I wanted to test for an interaction between age and GPA, to establish whether the association between GPA differed for different ages at onset. As with the other disorders, I also wanted to stratify by sex and look for an interaction with sex, since most similar studies have used males only.

Parental education level was strongly associated with school performance and with risk for bipolar disorder, such that better parental education was associated with increased risk for bipolar disorder. However, in contrast to the other two disorders, school performance has a U-shaped association with risk for bipolar, so it was possible that parental education would act as a confounder at higher levels of school performance, and a negative confounder at the lower end. It was certainly important to explore the relationship between parental education, school performance and risk for bipolar disorder.

Low head circumference and preterm delivery were both associated with poor school performance and risk for bipolar, so I wished to test whether these were acting as confounders.

Paternal age was associated with increased risk for bipolar, but had only a weak association with school performance, so it was unlikely to have a major effect, but I wished to confirm this.

Bipolar disorder – results

Although confounding was somewhat more important in bipolar than the other disorders, the fully adjusted model (Table 6.15), had essentially the same pattern of findings as the unadjusted model.

Pupils with excellent school performance (2 standard deviations above the population mean) had an approximately threefold risk of bipolar

TABLE 6.15
Hazard ratios for bipolar disorder, controlling for parental
education, preterm delivery and head circumference

Parameter	Hazard ratio	p>z	95% confidence interval
GPA Z-score			
Below −2	2.13	0.010	1.20 to 3.78
−2 to −1	1.33	0.119	0.93 to 1.91
−1 to +1 (ref)	1.00	–	– –
+1 to +2	1.31	0.117	0.94 to 1.82
Over +2	2.98	0.001	1.56 to 5.70
Parental education			
Parental education 1	0.85	0.528	0.51 to 1.41
Parental education 2	0.92	0.680	0.62 to 1.36
Parental education 4	1.14	0.551	0.74 to 1.76
Parental education 5	1.50	0.040	1.02 to 2.21
Preterm delivery	2.10	0.002	1.31 to 3.34
Head circumference			
Low head circumference	1.80	0.027	1.07 to 3.03
High head circumference	0.72	0.517	0.27 to 1.94

GPA, grade-point average.

disorder, and, although this was partially confounded by parental education, it remained significant after controlling for parental education.

Pupils with very poor performance (2 standard deviations below the population mean) were at around a twofold increased risk for bipolar disorder. There was some negative confounding by parental education, such that, when parental education was added to the model, the association strengthened.

There was weak evidence that the association with low scores may have been confounded by head circumference and preterm delivery.

The association with high scores appeared more marked in males, whereas the association with low scores appeared more marked in females, but this may have been an artefact, and there was no statistical evidence of any interaction between school performance and gender.

CHAPTER SEVEN

School performance in individual school subjects

ANALYSIS STRATEGY

In the previous four chapters, I have demonstrated clear associations between overall grade-point average (GPA) and risk for schizophrenia, schizoaffective disorder and bipolar disorder. The purpose of this chapter is to establish whether these associations apply across all school subjects, or whether particular subjects are more important than others.

Grades ranged from A to E for each school subject, so I used E grade as the exposure, and grades B–D as the reference category. In the case of English and mathematics, which are streamed, I used two exposure variables: being in the lower stream, and having an E grade. In the case of bipolar disorder, where high, as well as low grades may be a risk factor, I repeated the analysis, using grade A as the exposure.

I began by examining E grades in each school subject as individual risk factors, by performing separate, unadjusted regression analyses for each school subject. However, particularly in the case of schizophrenia, the relative contributions of specific school subjects were difficult to differentiate because of the strength of the generalised deficit. I therefore performed adjusted analyses, in which all the school subjects are included the same model, so that the hazard ratio (HR) for an E grade in each subject is adjusted for E grades in all other subjects. This allowed me to determine which subjects were contributing most strongly to the overall association with GPA. Many of the subjects had a strong bias in favour of one or other gender (data not shown). I therefore also controlled for sex in the adjusted analysis.

I will present the school subjects in order of the strength of their effects (in order of decreasing hazard ratio in the adjusted analysis).

SCHIZOPHRENIA

Table 7.1 and Figure 7.1 show the hazard ratios for schizophrenia, with E grades in each subject as the exposure. In the case of mathematics and English, both of which were streamed, being in the lower stream is also included as an exposure.

The left column of Table 7.1 shows unadjusted hazard ratios for scoring an E grade, or being in the lower stream, of each subject. The right hand column shows the hazard ratios adjusted for E grade in all other subjects, and for sex. This allows us to discern the relative strength of the risk factors compared with the others. To understand the interpretation of the data, take music as an example. The unadjusted HR is 2.54, meaning that scoring an E grade in music is associated with an increase in hazard of schizophrenia by around 2.5 times. The adjusted HR, however, is 1.00. This means that, after taking into account information on the E grades in all other subjects, as well as sex differences, having an E grade in music has no additional effect on risk for schizophrenia. In other words, one's perform-ance in music is about averagely predictive of schizophrenia, when com-pared with one's performance in the other subjects and one's sex. Subjects higher in the list, such as engineering, tend to have a stronger relationship, and subjects below 1.00 have a weaker effect. But despite having hazard ratios less than 1, they are certainly not protective against schizophrenia.

It is very striking that, without exception, scoring grade E or being in the lower stream is a strong risk factor for schizophrenia. E grades in engineering, civics or biology, and being in the lower stream in mathematics were all significant predictors of schizophrenia even after adjusting for all other subjects and sex, although there is no particular logic in focusing on the p-values in the adjusted analysis; all subjects are strongly predictive of schizophrenia, and in the adjusted analysis we are only looking at their relative strength. Although there is no strong pattern, there is a general tendency for mathematical and scientific subjects to be stronger predictors of schizophrenia than the humanities.

SCHIZOAFFECTIVE DISORDER

For schizoaffective disorder, I conducted an identical analysis. The results are shown in Table 7.2 and Figure 7.1.

In the unadjusted analysis, over half the school subjects were signi-ficantly associated with risk for schizoaffective disorder, and even in those

TABLE 7.1
Hazard ratios (HRs) for schizophrenia, by E grades in each school subject

Subject	Unadjusted			Adjusted		
	HR	p<Z	95% CI	HR	p<Z	95% CI
Engineering	4.33	<0.001	2.99 to 6.27	1.99	0.004	1.25 to 3.18
Civics	3.16	<0.001	2.32 to 4.31	1.85	0.014	1.13 to 3.01
Biology	3.57	<0.001	2.65 to 4.82	1.63	0.035	1.03 to 2.57
Maths (low stream)	1.70	<0.001	1.43 to 2.04	1.43	0.001	1.15 to 1.78
Sports	2.52	<0.001	1.78 to 3.57	1.42	0.084	0.95 to 2.11
Maths (E)	1.70	<0.001	1.43 to 2.04	1.39	0.147	0.89 to 2.16
Art	3.29	<0.001	2.14 to 5.03	1.35	0.229	0.83 to 2.22
Chemistry	2.96	<0.001	2.23 to 3.92	1.25	0.326	0.80 to 1.94
Home economics	3.05	<0.001	1.97 to 4.72	1.14	0.628	0.68 to 1.90
Swedish	3.09	<0.001	2.08 to 4.58	1.12	0.667	0.67 to 1.85
English (low stream)	1.60	<0.001	1.34 to 1.91	1.04	0.728	0.83 to 1.30
Music	2.54	<0.001	1.64 to 3.94	1.00	0.997	0.61 to 1.64
English (E)	2.39	<0.001	1.54 to 3.70	0.97	0.899	0.59 to 1.60
Physics	2.73	<0.001	2.01 to 3.70	0.93	0.752	0.58 to 1.48
Geography	2.57	<0.001	1.80 to 3.66	0.91	0.725	0.54 to 1.53
Handicrafts	2.57	<0.001	1.48 to 4.46	0.91	0.755	0.49 to 1.67
History	2.31	<0.001	1.65 to 3.25	0.80	0.394	0.47 to 1.34
Childcare	1.97	<0.001	1.36 to 2.84	0.69	0.095	0.44 to 1.07
Religion	2.29	<0.001	1.62 to 3.23	0.69	0.168	0.41 to 1.17
(Female sex)	–	–	–	0.56	<0.001	0.46 to 0.68

Adjusted HRs are adjusted for each other, and for sex. The reference category comprises pupils scoring B–D. CI, confidence interval.

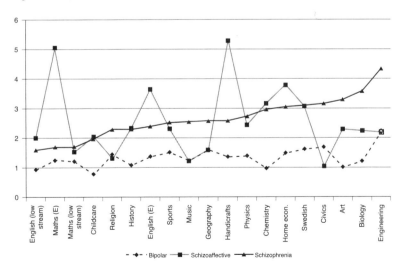

Figure 7.1 Unadjusted hazard ratios for E grades in each school subject. The school subjects are arranged along the x-axis in order of increasing assocation with schizophrenia

TABLE 7.2
Hazard ratios (HRs) for schizoaffective disorder, by E grades in each school subject

Subject	Unadjusted			Adjusted		
	HR	*p<Z*	*95% CI*	*HR*	*p<Z*	*95% CI*
Maths	5.05	<0.001	2.62 to 9.73	3.39	0.003	1.50 to 7.69
Handicrafts	5.29	<0.001	2.15 to 13.02	2.77	0.060	0.96 to 7.99
Chemistry	3.16	<0.001	1.68 to 5.92	2.03	0.131	0.81 to 5.09
English	3.63	0.002	1.59 to 8.31	1.96	0.179	0.73 to 5.24
Home economics	3.82	0.004	1.55 to 9.40	1.92	0.242	0.64 to 5.72
History	2.34	0.030	1.08 to 5.06	1.92	0.228	0.66 to 5.56
English (low stream)	2.00	0.001	1.34 to 3.00	1.76	0.028	1.06 to 2.90
Swedish	3.09	0.014	1.25 to 7.60	1.29	0.655	0.42 to 3.99
Sports	2.30	0.049	1.00 to 5.26	1.19	0.717	0.47 to 3.01
Maths (low stream)	1.53	0.039	1.02 to 2.30	0.99	0.978	0.60 to 1.64
Art	2.29	0.156	0.73 to 7.26	0.95	0.939	0.26 to 3.44
Childcare	2.05	0.089	0.90 to 4.69	0.93	0.884	0.35 to 2.49
Physics	2.44	0.016	1.18 to 5.04	0.91	0.858	0.33 to 2.54
Biology	2.24	0.056	0.98 to 5.12	0.79	0.673	0.26 to 2.38
Engineering	2.18	0.183	0.69 to 6.90	0.74	0.657	0.20 to 2.75
Geography	1.58	0.373	0.58 to 4.29	0.70	0.588	0.19 to 2.55
Music	1.23	0.770	0.30 to 5.00	0.43	0.274	0.10 to 1.95
Religion	1.31	0.588	0.48 to 3.59	0.43	0.217	0.12 to 1.63
Civics	1.05	0.927	0.33 to 3.33	0.29	0.096	0.07 to 1.25
(Female sex)	–	–	– –	1.04	0.838	0.69 to 1.59

Adjusted HRs are adjusted for each other, and for sex. The reference category comprises pupils scoring B–D. CI, confidence interval.

which were not significant, risk was higher for students with E grades than those without, in every subject. In comparing the p-values to those for schizophrenia, it is important to note that there were fewer individuals with schizoaffective disorder, giving less statistical power, and most of the hazard ratios are in a similar range to those of schizophrenia.

Looking at the adjusted results, however, one can see that the subjects that contribute the greatest risk for schizoaffective disorder are quite different than those for schizophrenia. This is best seen in Figure 7.1. Many subjects, such as engineering and civics, seem to have rather different associations with schizophrenia and schizoaffective disorder. The slight tendency for scientific subjects to have a stronger association with schizophrenia than non-scientific subjects does not seem to be present for schizoaffective disorder.

BIPOLAR DISORDER

For bipolar disorder, I began by performing the same analysis as for the other two disorders (Table 7.3 and Figure 7.1).

TABLE 7.3
Hazard ratios (HRs) for bipolar disorder, by E grades in each school subject

Subject	Unadjusted			Adjusted		
	HR	p<Z	95% CI	HR	p<Z	95% CI
Engineering E	2.22	0.019	1.41 to 4.31	2.11	0.069	0.94 to 4.71
Swedish E	1.63	0.174	0.81 to 3.29	1.44	0.414	0.60 to 3.49
Geography E	1.60	0.111	0.90 to 2.85	1.37	0.468	0.59 to 3.20
Maths (low stream)	1.22	0.099	0.96 to 1.54	1.30	0.066	0.98 to 1.71
Home economics E	1.50	0.326	0.67 to 3.37	1.29	0.593	0.51 to 3.26
Religion E	1.45	0.187	0.83 to 2.54	1.28	0.567	0.55 to 2.98
Sports E	1.52	0.155	0.85 to 2.71	1.27	0.459	0.67 to 2.42
Physics E	1.40	0.226	0.81 to 2.39	1.20	0.629	0.57 to 2.55
English E	1.38	0.404	0.65 to 2.91	1.08	0.867	0.46 to 2.51
Music E	1.25	0.588	0.56 to 2.81	1.03	0.957	0.42 to 2.52
Handicrafts E	1.37	0.53	0.51 to 1.70	1.00	0.994	0.34 to 2.93
Chemistry E	0.98	0.951	0.54 to 1.79	0.56	0.171	0.24 to 1.28
Childcare E	0.78	0.510	0.37 to 1.65	0.55	0.171	0.24 to 1.29
History E	1.09	0.798	0.58 to 2.04	0.51	0.153	0.20 to 1.28
Civics E	1.70	0.054	0.99 to 2.91	1.75	0.183	0.77 to 3.99
Art E	1.02	0.971	0.38 to 2.73	0.77	0.637	0.26 to 2.26
English (low stream)	0.94	0.658	0.73 to 1.22	0.80	0.153	0.59 to 1.09
Maths E	1.26	0.542	0.62 to 2.54	0.99	0.984	0.44 to 2.22
Biology E	1.22	0.528	0.65 to 2.30	0.96	0.928	0.41 to 2.26
(Female sex)	–	–	– –	1.18	0.171	0.93 to 1.51

Adjusted HRs are adjusted for each other, and for sex. The reference category comprises pupils scoring B–D. CI, confidence interval.

E grades in most subjects had little or no association with risk for bipolar disorder. The only subject in which an E grade significantly predicted bipolar was engineering.

Table 7.4 shows the equivalent analysis, but using grade A as the exposure. The unadjusted analysis shows that individuals with A grades in music, childcare, biology, geography, Swedish, religion, history, home economics, English, civics and history had higher rates of bipolar disorder. Maths and engineering were almost significant, despite E grades in the latter also being associated with bipolar disorder. A grades in sports and handicrafts were protective against bipolar.

CONCLUSIONS

In this chapter, I assessed the contributions of different school subjects to the associations with GPA that I had described in earlier chapters. E grades were associated with two- to fourfold increases in risk for schizophrenia, which were significant at the p<0.001 level in all school subjects. When each

TABLE 7.4

Hazard ratios (HRs) for bipolar disorder, by A grades in each school subject

Subject	Unadjusted					Adjusted	
	HR	p<Z	95% CI	HR	p<Z	95% CI	
Music A	2.07	<0.001	1.50 to 2.88	1.65	0.007	1.15 to 2.36	
Childcare A	2.22	<0.001	1.60 to 3.07	1.61	0.020	1.08 to 2.42	
Biology A	2.03	<0.001	1.47 to 2.81	1.54	0.079	0.95 to 2.50	
Geography A	2.12	<0.001	1.53 to 2.97	1.49	0.119	0.90 to 2.47	
Swedish A	2.26	<0.001	1.60 to 3.19	1.42	0.144	0.89 to 2.28	
Engineering A	1.60	0.068	0.97 to 2.65	1.29	0.380	0.73 to 2.28	
Religion A	2.02	<0.001	1.45 to 2.80	1.16	0.566	0.70 to 1.92	
Maths A	1.44	0.062	0.98 to 2.12	1.09	0.715	0.69 to 1.72	
Home economics A	1.69	0.007	1.15 to 2.48	1.07	0.782	0.68 to 1.68	
Art A	1.38	0.017	0.93 to 2.04	1.05	0.817	0.69 to 1.59	
History A	1.86	<0.001	1.33 to 2.57	1.05	0.862	0.63 to 1.75	
English A	1.61	0.015	1.09 to 2.36	0.92	0.738	0.58 to 1.47	
Civics A	1.73	0.002	1.23 to 2.45	0.86	0.562	0.51 to 1.44	
Chemistry A	1.53	0.023	1.06 to 2.19	0.83	0.491	0.49 to 1.41	
Physics A	1.31	0.171	0.89 to 1.92	0.64	0.106	0.37 to 1.10	
Handicrafts A	0.65	0.139	0.36 to 1.15	0.46	0.012	0.25 to 0.84	
Sports A	0.42	0.004	0.24 to 0.75	0.38	0.001	0.21 to 0.67	
(Female sex)	–	–	– –.	1.01	0.953	0.78 to 1.30	

Adjusted HRs are adjusted for each other, and for sex. The reference category comprises pupils scoring B–D. CI, confidence interval.

school subject was controlled for performance in all other subjects, science and mathematics seemed to have the strongest associations.

In schizoaffective disorder, hazard ratios for E grades were in the same range, although not all were statistically significant, due to lower power. Poor scores in mathematics were again strongly associated with disease, but the pattern was not clearly similar to that in schizophrenia.

Poor performance in mathematics and engineering was modestly associated with bipolar disorder, but A grades in several predominantly arts subjects were associated with around a doubling in risk for bipolar disorder.

CHAPTER EIGHT

General discussion

SUMMARY OF FINDINGS

In this study, I have used data spanning a 30-year period from almost a million individuals to investigate the association between school performance at age 16 and risk for psychotic disorders up to age 30, using a population cohort covering the whole of Sweden, controlling for potential confounders. The principal findings were as follows.

1. School performance followed a bell-shaped distribution, with risk for mental disorders concentrated in upper and lower extremes of the curve.
2. Poor school performance is a strong risk factor for both schizophrenia and schizoaffective disorder, and a weaker risk factor for bipolar affective disorder.
3. Excellent school performance in protective against both schizophrenia and schizoaffective disorder.
4. Excellent school performance is a risk factor for bipolar affective disorder.
5. There is little or no confounding by migration, socioeconomic group, parental education, pregnancy and birth characteristics, parental age at birth, season of birth, birth order or family size.

6. The association between poor school performance and schizophrenia is present independently in all compulsory school subjects studied, with a tendency towards especially poor performance in mathematical and scientific subjects.
7. The association between excellent school performance and bipolar disorder is present in most school subjects, particularly in arts/humanities subjects.

STRENGTHS AND WEAKNESSES OF THIS RESEARCH

Bias

Selection bias

Selection bias is a sampling error whereby the probability of inclusion in the sample is related to exposure and/or outcome, leading to a biased estimate of the association between exposure and outcome. It is generally more of a problem in case–control and intervention studies than in cohort studies. Furthermore, one of the major strengths of population-based cohort studies such as this one, is that the sample is close to 100% of the target population, leaving little scope for selection bias.

Several of the most impressive prospective studies in this field have used military conscription data, but some of these suffered from potential selection biases: there were often no data for females, and individuals who were excused conscription were typically excluded. Our sample, in contrast, included every child leaving compulsory school from the whole of Sweden over a 9-year period.

It is not possible to determine how many children in Sweden do not undergo compulsory schooling, but the number is likely to be very low. According to *Skolverket* (the Swedish national agency for education) the percentage of compulsory school children registered with learning disabilities in 2002/3 (the only year for which I have been able to obtain information) was 1.4%. Some of these children would not have been included in the sample, leading to a sample containing fewer poor performers. This may have led to a slight underestimate of the association between low performance and psychosis.

Less than 0.1% of children were in special schools for sensory impairments, and although I have not been able to ascertain whether they were included in the register, their numbers are so small that it is unlikely this would have greatly affected the results. Private schools, which were very uncommon, were obliged to follow the same curriculum and examinations as state schools and were also included in the registers.

Information bias

Information bias is a systematic error in measuring exposure or disease status.

Loss to follow-up

A major source of information bias in cohort studies is loss to follow-up, whereby patients that are followed up differ systematically from those who are not followed up, or those followed for longer differ from those followed for less time. The purpose of the survival analysis that I used was to adjust for this type of bias. However, in practice, similar results were obtained whether or not censoring was taken into account.

Misclassification of exposure and reverse causality

One of the main advantages of prospective study designs is that disease outcome cannot bias the measurement of the exposure, since the exposure is measured before the onset of the disorder. However, this assumes that the timing of onset is accurate. The age at onset of psychosis is notoriously difficult to ascertain, and this study relied on the relatively crude indicator of hospital admission. It is likely that some individuals were suffering from prodromal or even actual symptoms of psychosis at the time that they took their examinations (albeit not sufficiently severe to warrant their being excused from the examinations or admitted to hospital) and that this might have influenced their performance. This is referred to as reverse causality bias.

I took two steps to try to minimise reverse causality bias. First, I excluded any children who had an admission prior to their examinations. Second, I also excluded admissions in the first year after taking the examinations, so that children who were in the early or prodromal stages of psychosis when they took their examinations would not bias the results in favour of poor performance. Nevertheless, prodromal symptoms lasting more than a year before first admission could have biased the results.

If a large proportion of individuals had performed poorly as a direct result of prodromal psychosis, one would expect to see worse school performance in earlier onset patients, but there was no strong evidence of this (Figures 5.8, 5.12, 5.14, 5.15, 5.16, 5.18).

Given the observed association between excellent school performance and bipolar disorder, it is conceivable that students with prodromal symptoms of mania might actually perform *better* than average. Clearly, full mania is likely to impair performance, but it is possible that subclinical hypomanic symptoms may have enabled pupils to work harder or faster (discussed in greater detail on page 138). If this were the case, we would

expect to see an association between early age at onset and school performance. Figure 5.18 shows no strong association over the whole range of
school performance. On the other hand, the greatest risk of bipolar disorder
is associated with excellent (>+2 SD) school performance. Figure 5.16
shows that students with excellent school performance did tend to have
earlier onsets, which suggests that reverse causality might be operating, at
least in the highest category of school performance.

Misclassification of outcome

In common with most other Western countries, Swedish psychiatric care is
increasingly delivered in community, rather than hospital, settings. Some
patients with psychosis would undoubtedly have remained well enough not
to require hospitalisation during the course of the study, which would have
biased the sample to include more severe cases. This would have included
some patients who were not in contact with the mental health services at all,
and almost by definition, it is difficult to estimate their numbers.

Two studies have addressed the effects of the introduction of community
care on hospitalisation rates in Sweden. In a 4-year comparison before and
after the introduction of sectorised community services in a Swedish
catchment area in the 1980s, Hansson found that the length of admissions
decreased by about 40%, and the number of admissions per patient by 20%,
but there was almost no reduction in the total number of patients hospitalised (Hansson, 1989). A more recent study, conducted between 1994 and
2003 (i.e. concurrently with this study) had very similar findings: although
the total number of days spent in psychiatric beds fell dramatically, the
number of patients admitted scarcely changed (Arvidsson & Ericson, 2005).
These studies provide some reassurance that the proportion of individuals
with psychosis misclassified as unaffected is probably not increasing
significantly, but unfortunately there are very few data on the likely base-
line rate of non-admitted psychosis. We can be certain that our sample is
biased towards more severe cases, but the extent of the bias is difficult to
estimate.

The effect of non-admission may bias the results differently depending
on the diagnostic group. Again, it is difficult to predict which way these
biases might operate. For example, bipolar disorder is usually associated
with less social deterioration than schizophrenia, so one might expect any
bias due to non-admission to be more severe with bipolar disorder than
schizophrenia. On the other hand, patients with a first onset of schizophrenia are often withdrawn and apathetic, and may not complain of
feeling unwell. Individuals with mania, however, might be more likely to
behave in reckless, aggressive or inappropriate ways that bring them to the
attention of mental health services.

The effect of this bias towards severe cases on the association between school performance and psychosis depends on whether school performance is related to the probability of admission. If school performance were unrelated to the probability of a patient with psychosis being admitted, then a random assortment of the true cases of psychosis would be misclassified as unaffected (non-differential misclassification). This noise in the data would, on average, have the effect of reducing the size of the effect.

If individuals with psychosis and poor school grades are more likely to be admitted than those with average school grades, then the individuals who were not admitted (i.e. who were misclassified as unaffected) would tend to be better performers (differential misclassification). This type of bias would have the effect of increasing the estimate of the association between poor performance and psychosis, while reducing the estimate of the association between good performance and psychosis.

Cognitive ability might well influence the probability of admission. It is likely that more intelligent individuals would be more successful at concealing or downplaying their symptoms than less intelligent ones. Again, this effect might operate differently in schizophrenia versus bipolar disorder. In schizophrenia, it is possible to harbour delusions and experience hallucinations without necessarily behaving abnormally, and most patients have limited insight into their illness, especially in the first episode, and may therefore try to evade treatment. Secondary abnormal behaviour, which might lead to admission, might be subject to greater individual control in people with higher cognitive ability. In mania however, the syndrome is, to a considerable extent, defined by behaviour. Even the most intelligent patient would find it difficult to contain the symptoms of mania, and most patients with bipolar depression will actively seek help rather than try to conceal their symptoms.

We can obtain indirect evidence as to whether patients with worse school grades are more likely to be admitted. If poor school performance were associated with increased probability of admission, then it might follow that patients with lower grades would have more admissions. Figure 6.4 on page 103 shows that there is no association between number of admissions and grade-point average (GPA) for any diagnosis (no correlations significant at the $p=0.05$ level). This suggests that any misclassification of the outcome is likely to be non-differential, so any bias will be towards the null, i.e. in the direction of no effect.

Observer bias

Observer bias generally refers to bias on the part of the experimenter, but in this study, the experimenter had no direct interaction with the subjects. The exposure and outcome were both assessed by third parties: (teachers in the case of the exposure, and psychiatrists in the case of the outcome). As discussed in the methods section, teachers had only limited powers to increase or decrease the grade of the children, and it is difficult to imagine how their assessments could have been biased, since they had no knowledge of the outcome. However, there is a possibility that the psychiatrists who made the diagnoses could have been biased by knowledge of their patients' school grades. For example, anecdotal evidence suggests that some psychiatrists may be more inclined to assign a diagnosis of bipolar disorder to an intelligent patient, but schizoaffective disorder or schizophrenia to a patient with poor cognitive function (personal communications with various psychiatrists, referees' comments during peer review).

Confounding

Measured

Measured confounding refers to confounding by variables that are measured. The main methods of controlling for measured confounding are by matching (in case–control studies), by controlling for the potential confounders in the analysis or by restriction (excluding individuals with a potential confounding factor).

I chose the method of restriction in the case of migrants, both first and second generation, because migrant status is likely to be a confounder in studies of this type, since migrants are at increased risk for schizophrenia (Cantor-Graae & Selten, 2005) and also tend to perform poorly at school (Gonzalez, 2003). Furthermore, much of the missing data for the parents related to parents who were born outside Sweden, so by excluding them I was able to reduce the amount of missing data to very low levels, typically 0.5% (see Table 5.4).

I was able to adjust for a range of other potential confounders, which I selected a priori on the basis that they were likely to be associated with both school performance and psychosis, including birth characteristics, parental age, parental education level, socioeconomic status and spring birth. I have listed the details of which associations were confounded by which variables (see Chapters 5–7). Overall, there was surprisingly little confounding by any of the measured variables. The association between school performance and schizophrenia was confounded to some extent by sex, socioeconomic group and family size, although the association remained strong even after adjusting for these confounders. The associations in bipolar disorder were partially confounded by parental education, but remained significant after controlling for parental education, and there was weak evidence that the association with low scores may have been confounded by head circumference and preterm delivery in the case of bipolar disorder.

Residual

Residual confounding is confounding by factors that were measured to some extent, but not sufficiently accurately or finely to reduce or abolish the association between exposure and outcome. It is certainly possible that we had residual confounding in this study. Some of the variables that I used in trying to adjust for confounding were relatively crude. For example, socio-economic group was measured on a six-point scale by parental occupation. It is quite likely that socioeconomic factors related to deprivation could have been confounding the association, but may not have been captured by a simple measure of socioeconomic status. If one were to design a traditional cohort study, based on questionnaires, one would aim to collect much more detailed information about social circumstances, family dynamics, economic deprivation, social capital, and the mental health of parents and carers. Any of these factors may be confounding the associations, leading to residual and unmeasured confounding.

Unmeasured

Unmeasured confounding is confounding by factors that are not measured. By definition it is impossible to detect or control for unmeasured confounding, so one can only speculate as to possible unmeasured confounders. One possible unmeasured confounder is mental disorder in the parents. Around 10% of Swedish individuals with schizophrenia have a parent with schizophrenia (Lichtenstein et al., 2006). If having a parent with schizophrenia leads to impaired school performance (one can imagine plausible genetic and environmental mechanisms for such an association), then this could account for some or all of the observed association between poor performance and schizophrenia. Personality and social factors may also be acting as unmeasured confounders. For example, a socially withdrawn or paranoid personality could lead to underachievement at school and also be independently associated with risk for psychosis.

Use of registers for diagnoses

The Swedish population registers are very carefully collected and maintained. However, the study relies on the accuracy and validity of the data within the registers, particularly the validity of diagnoses in the register. There are two main concerns: that Swedish diagnostic practice may be different to that in other countries, and that it may be inconsistent even within Sweden.

Dalman and colleagues (2002) addressed both these concerns with respect to schizophrenia. The authors randomly selected 100 cases of schizophrenia from the registries and diagnosed them according to DSM–IV (even though the registers are coded using ICD–10). In all 86% fulfilled the DSM–IV criteria of 'schizophrenia syndrome' (codes 295.1–4, 295.6–7, 295.9) and 76% fulfilled the 'narrow' definition of schizophrenia in DSM–IV (which excluded schizoaffective disorder, borderline schizophrenia and schizophreniform disorder) (Dalman et al., 2002). They also found good temporal stability and minimal differences in the reliability of diagnoses between regions. Ekholm and colleagues (2005) performed a similar study using a clinically selected sample, and found an almost identical positive predictive value of 75% for a register diagnosis of schizophrenia, against a gold standard of interview and case-note assessment by an experienced psychiatrist using DSM–IV criteria. In the latter study, the kappa value for agreement between register and diagnostic interview-based diagnoses was worryingly low at around 0.3. However, this low value was largely because 41% of cases diagnosed in the register as having other psychotic disorders (most of whom would be classified under 'other psychoses' in my sample) were judged to have DSM–IV schizophrenia at interview. This suggests that Swedish psychiatrists were employing a more conservative definition of schizophrenia than that of DSM–IV. I would expect that higher rates of agreement would have been demonstrated in both studies had the researchers used ICD criteria rather than DSM criteria as their 'gold standard', since the registers use ICD categories.

I have not been able to find any similar data on the diagnostic validity of bipolar disorder.

COMPARISON WITH OTHER STUDIES

Schizophrenia

My results concord with almost all other studies by showing pre-morbid cognitive deficits in psychosis. The two Finnish studies that used school grades (Isohanni et al., 1998; Cannon et al., 1999) were the only ones not to find a substantial deficit in children who went on to develop schizophrenia. This was thought perhaps to be because educational attainment was a poor indicator of cognitive functioning, but my results suggest that educational attainment is a strong predictor of later psychosis.

How can we explain the discrepancy between these results? Cannon and colleagues (1999) have pointed out that the Finnish school system during the period of their study was very structured and supportive, with a strong emphasis on preventing children from falling behind. However, the Swedish education system appears to share these characteristics (Sven Sundin (of the Swedish Education department, *Skolverket*), personal communication).

Individuals who went on to develop schizophrenia in the Helsinki cohort, despite having similar scores, were less likely than their peers to progress to upper secondary school education (Cannon et al., 1999), suggesting that there were some shortcomings in their school performance, which may not have been captured in their school grades. It is also notable that the Helsinki study examined school performance at a relatively early age, and there is some evidence from the British (Jones et al., 1994) and Israeli (Reichenberg et al., 2005) studies that deficits are greater at later ages. There were also missing school data on over half the schizophrenia cases in the Helsinki study, and it is possible that this may have biased the results.

The lack of an association with school grades in the North Finland 1966 study is also difficult to explain, although, like the Helsinki study, there was circumstantial evidence of poor performance in children who went on to develop schizophrenia compared with their classmates; they were more often below their expected grades in class at age 14 (Isohanni et al., 1999).

In both studies, it is unclear whether any procedures were in place for standardising and peer-referencing school grades in Finland in the 1960s and 1970s. If such procedures existed at all, they may not have been as rigorous and sophisticated as those in Sweden in the 1990s, as described on page 51.

There is one other puzzling aspect of Finland that may be relevant. It appears that there were few or no cases of bipolar disorder, at least in the 1966 North Finland cohort (bipolar disorder was not considered in the Helsinki study so it is not clear whether any cases existed or not). The authors of the North Finland study describe in some detail the categorisation of psychiatric disorders into four groups: (1) schizophrenia; (2) other psychoses; (3) non-psychotic disorders; and (4) no psychiatric disorder, and list the main ICD codes included in each category. Neither bipolar disorder, nor its code (code 296.x in ICD–9) is mentioned, which suggests that few or no cases were found.

This is consistent with previous research demonstrating that bipolar disorder appears to be exceedingly rare in Finland, and the few cases that do exist have a very late peak onset of 50–59 years (Rasanen et al., 1998). In young adults, the incidence rate is about a tenth of that reported in comparable studies in other countries (Rasanen et al., 1998).

Why are these rates so low? Two explanations are possible. One possibility is that the training or diagnostic tradition of Finnish psychiatrists is atypical, and patients presenting with symptoms characteristic of bipolar disorder are less likely to attract a diagnosis of bipolar disorder in Finland than in most other countries. The second possibility is that the true prevalence of bipolar disorder is smaller in Finland.

The Finnish population is thought to be descended from a small number of ancestral founders, and to have been relatively isolated (Norio, 2003). Due to founder effects and subsequent genetic drift, over 30 rare genetic disorders have been described that seem to exist only in Finland, and some other genetic disorders (such as phenylketonuria and cystic fibrosis) are relatively common in other Caucasian populations, but rare or unknown in Finland (Norio, 2003). Bipolar disorder is almost certainly a polygenic disorder, so its low prevalence is unlikely to be explained by the absence of a particular allele, but the relative genetic isolation of Finland may still be relevant.

One highly speculative but intriguing possibility is that, in the context of the Finnish genetic background, genes that would predispose to bipolar disorder in most countries predispose instead to a phenotype that is indistinguishable from schizophrenia in Finnish populations. This could explain why Finnish schizophrenia cases appear less cognitively impaired than the schizophrenia cases identified in Sweden. It might also explain why excellent school performance is associated with schizophrenia in the Finnish sample, but with bipolar in the Swedish sample. However, I must emphasise that this suggestion is very speculative.

Bipolar disorder

To my knowledge, only four previous prospective population-based studies (Cannon et al., 2002b; Reichenberg et al., 2002; Zammit et al., 2004; Tiihonen et al., 2005) have examined pre-morbid cognitive functioning in bipolar disorder, and none have used school records. None of them have found significant pre-morbid deficits in bipolar disorder.

Our results showed a U-shaped relationship between school performance and risk for bipolar (Figure 5.18). The U-shaped association that we found is only discernable if school performance is divided into several categories. Simply comparing means, as was done in the Israeli and Dunedin studies, would not capture the effect. After seeing our results, my colleague Avi Reichenberg re-analysed data from the Israeli cohorts, using high performance as an exposure, and obtained results similar to mine, with a U-shaped relationship between cognitive abilities and risk for bipolar in several cognitive domains (Avi Reichenberg, personal communication). The other two studies (Zammit et al., 2004; Tiihonen et al., 2005) did divide performance into categories, but neither found strong evidence of a U-shaped association.

Superior pre-morbid functioning in bipolar disorder has been noted in some previous studies. Cannon and colleagues examined prospectively collected data on pre-morbid cognitive and neuromotor development in children who went on to develop mania (Cannon et al., 2002b). Although individuals who went on to develop mania did not differ from controls on cognitive measures, they performed significantly better than controls on motor performance, even after controlling for sex and socioeconomic status. Very recently, the same researchers showed that these children who went on to develop mania also had significantly higher IQs than the remainder of the cohort, but the authors acknowledged that the sample was small, with only 8 children who went on to develop mania, and they called for replications in a larger sample (Koenen et al., 2009).

McIntosh and colleagues (2005) found that bipolar patients from multiply-affected families scored higher than their unaffected relatives on the National Adult Reading Test (a measure of pre-morbid intelligence). Kutcher and colleagues (1998), applying *a priori* criteria to prospectively collected school records, found that 68% of 28 adolescent-onset bipolar I patients had 'good/excellent' pre-morbid academic function, whereas only 30% were judged to have excellent pre-morbid social functioning. Lastly, Aro and colleagues, in a population-based Finnish study found higher admission rates for bipolar disorder in people who had completed more than 12 years of education, whereas the reverse was true for other psychotic and affective disorders (Aro et al., 1995).

INTERPRETATION OF FINDINGS

School performance versus cognitive functioning

The use of school performance as measured by this study (see page 51), raises two questions: what is the relationship between school performance, traditional measures of neuropsychological function and intelligence, and does GPA represent absolute or relative performance?

What is the relationship between school performance, neuropsychological function and intelligence?

Cognitive tests are generally considered to be the most objective measures of intellectual function because they are, ideally, administered and scored in a standardised way. School performance is traditionally seen as less objective and more subject to random variations and systematic biases than neuropsychological tests. Scores on neuropsychological tests are often seen as a gold standard against which other measures of ability should be measured. In particular, the concept of *g* is often regarded as the ultimate indicator of intelligence (see below).

It is probably true that school performance is a less direct measure of specific cognitive functions (such as verbal memory) than well-designed neurocognitive tests that are specifically designed to test these functions. Nevertheless, it is worth remembering that the rationale for the development of the first cognitive tests, such as the Stanford–Binet IQ tests, was to allow prediction of school performance (Deary et al., 2007), and cognitive tests were validated against educational outcomes, not the other way around.

A recent longitudinal study of 70,000 individuals showed that 50–60% of the variance in examination results at age 16 could be explained by intelligence at age 11 (Deary et al., 2007). Some of the residual variance will be attributable to measurement error, but the remainder is likely influenced by factors that are poorly captured by cognitive tests, such as long-term memory and attention, school attendance and engagement, motivation, diligence, organisational abilities, creativity and social competence. It has been argued that cognitive tests, with their emphasis on individual differences, measure a somewhat narrow range of abilities (Flynn, 2007).

What is g?

At the between-individuals level, all cognitive tests are correlated to some extent. In other words, if a panel of cognitive tests is administered to a set of individuals, subjects who score highly on any one test will tend to excel at the others; similarly, the poorest performers on a given test will tend to perform poorly across the board.

Factor analysis is a statistical technique in which the underlying correlation structure between several variables is examined. When the scores from a battery of tests are analysed using factor analysis, the correlations between individuals are condensed into statistical factors. g is simply the strongest factor to emerge from factor analysis; the one that explains the largest proportion of the inter-individual variability.

However, it is important to recognise that g is a statistical concept. It is not measured directly, and it correlates strongly with some tests but only weakly with others. It seems probable that it has some biological underpinnings, but our understanding of this is limited (Flynn, 2007) and attempts to find correlations of g with basic psychological processes such as reaction time have had mixed results (Deary, 2001; Deary & Crawford, 1998).

The psychologist James Flynn has criticised the concept of g as being a narrow assessment of intelligence that focuses too much on cross-sectional correlations at the level of individual differences. Crucially, factor analysis of cross-sectional data (on which g is based) is not capable of detecting the strong trend for IQ scores to improve from one generation to another, known as the Flynn effect (Flynn, 2007).

Several other authors have criticised the concept of g as being too narrow. Goleman (1995) argues that the underlying cognitive tests on which the concept of g rests are themselves constricted as they focus almost exclusively on reasoning and analytical thinking, often with a specific focus on scientific reasoning. He suggests that other qualities such as self-control, self-motivation and interpersonal skills, which he terms 'emotional intelligence', are equally important in predicting school grades and occupational success. Sternberg offers a tripartite model consisting of analytical, creative and practical intelligences, and presents preliminary evidence that his tests are superior to g in predicting real-world academic and occupational performance, including university GPAs (Sternberg, 1998; Sternberg et al., 2000).

We can conclude that our GPA score does not measure the same abilities as traditional cognitive tests, even if GPA is based on performance in a wide range of school subjects, and follows a similar bell-shaped distribution to g. From the evidence presented above, it is likely that GPA is moderately correlated with g. If g is considered the gold standard against which any other measure of performance should be judged, then GPA seems to be an imperfect measure. However, my view is that GPA is a *different* measure, but not necessarily any less valid. It may, if fact, be a better indicator of real-world functioning than the somewhat narrow concept of g.

Does GPA represent absolute or relative performance?

I will begin by answering the question: the effect of the elaborate system of norming is that GPA represents actual performance more closely than relative performance, despite the fact that it uses peer-referencing. However, the situation is complicated.

To recapitulate, the method used to calculate GPA was as follows: all school classes in Sweden were first graded against one another using the results of a small number of nationally standardised tests in key school subjects. The schools were thus ranked in terms of actual performance. The position of a school in the national ranking then determined the number of grades at A, B, C, D and E level that could be allocated to that class, and the allocation of grades within each class depended mainly on the performance of the pupil relative to his peers, but also to some extent on the subjective judgement of the teacher.

If the student's position within his own class was used on its own, the system would produce a relative measure of each person's performance against his peers, which could be taken as some indication of his ability in relation to others who had received a similar school environment. However, the additional step of allocating better or worse grades to each class depending on the ability of the whole class has the effect of peer-referencing students to the whole of Sweden rather than just their own class.

Under a relative system, a person who performed, for example, at exactly the fiftieth percentile within Sweden, might have received a B grade if he had attended a poorly performing school, but a D grade if he had attended a good school. His grade would be a reflection of his performance relative to his classmates. But under the system that was used, he should receive a C grade regardless of whether he attends the best-performing or the worst-performing school in Sweden, since his grade represents his performance relative to all the children in Sweden rather than just relative to his class. If he went to a very good school, he would be near the bottom of the class, but even pupils near the bottom of the class would receive C grades, rather than D or E grades, because the class would only have been allocated perhaps one or two D and E grades. Conversely, if the same pupil attended a very poorly performing school, he would be near the top of the class, but he would again receive a C grade because that class would have been allocated very few A or B grades. Of course, it is unlikely that the system worked perfectly, but in principle the GPA probably represents absolute performance more closely than relative (to the class) performance. Indeed, the system was designed to represent absolute performance. The aim was to produce a fair system such that all pupils in Sweden could compete on a level playing field for places in upper secondary school.

The association between low school performance and schizophrenia

A useful first step in interpreting any statistical association in epidemiology is to judge whether the association is spurious, indirect or causal (Grimes & Schulz, 2002). Spurious associations are a result of bias, confounding or chance. I have dealt with confounding and bias in previous sections, and concluded that these are unlikely to completely explain the association. The small p-values associated with the association indicate that it is very unlikely to be a chance finding. I have designed the study such that reverse causality, in its most literal sense of the outcome causing the exposure, is unlikely to explain the results. We are therefore left with the possibilities that the association is indirectly or directly causal.

A direct causal association refers to a cause–effect relationship between the exposure and outcome, in the sense that cigarette smoke has a direct effect on pulmonary tissue to increase the risk of cancer. It is scarcely credible that doing badly at school is itself a direct cause for schizophrenia. The only direct mechanism that I can conceive of would be that poor school grades produce psychosis by causing psychological stress.

An indirect association can be conceptualised as a type of confounding, where the exposure is a marker for one or more direct antecedents of the outcome, in the same way that socioeconomic group is a marker for some of the causes of heart disease. Most of the epidemiological risk factors for psychosis, such as poor school performance, urbanicity and migrant status are likely to fall into this category. So for what factors might school performance be a marker?

There are essentially three classes of mechanisms whereby poor school grades might be indirect risk markers for schizophrenia: biological, social and psychological. I will now consider each in turn.

Biological explanations

A biological explanation would see poor school grades as a marker of a physical abnormality in the brain. Given the weight of evidence for a neurodevelopmental aetiology of schizophrenia (see page 12), the most plausible biological explanation for the association is that poor school grades in individuals who go on to develop schizophrenia reflect neurodevelopmental impairment (Demjaha et al., in press).

Although it is certainly compatible with what we know about schizophrenia, the neurodevelopmental explanation raises further questions.

What is the biological basis of the neurodevelopmental problem inherent in schizophrenia: is it genetically or environmentally determined or both?

Unfortunately I have no data on genetic liability for schizophrenia, even at the crude level of family history. However, my results show that the association between school performance and schizophrenia does not seem to be related to the biological environmental factors that I have measured, particularly low birthweight, and hypoxia.

Do all patients with schizophrenia have some degree of neurodevelopmental impairment, or is there a specific neurodevelopmental subgroup?

Although poor school performance is associated with increased risk for schizophrenia, most schizophrenic patients have normal school performance. This pattern is found with many other risk indicators or correlates of schizophrenia. Might some patients have no neurodevelopmental impairment while a subgroup has a high degree of impairment?

If a neurodevelopmental subgroup were present that was associated with severe cognitive deficits, then one might detect a bimodal distribution in the scores of schizophrenic patients (Jones, 1995). There is no evidence for such a distribution (see Figure 5.13).

However, it seems more credible that neurodevelopmental problems will lead to a decrement in performance compared with an individual's expected performance, rather than causing low actual performance in every developmentally impaired individual. If this is the case, we should expect the school grades of individuals who go on to develop schizophrenia to be normally distributed, but with a lower mean than controls (Jones, 1995).

This is exactly the distribution that we observe: schizophrenia patients' scores follow a normal distribution, which is shifted downward (i.e. to the left) by around 0.5 standard deviations (Figure 5.13).

The distribution of scores cannot, however, tell us whether all individuals who go on to develop schizophrenia suffered a similar decrement, or whether some suffered large decrements, whereas others had no decrement. For example, the data would be equally compatible with all schizophrenic patients having a decrement of 0.5 standard deviations in their school performance, or with a neurodevelopmental subgroup having a 1 standard-deviation decrement, while a non-neurodevelopmental group suffered no decrement.

Is there more than one type of neurodevelopmental abnormality that can give rise to schizophrenia?

Given the diverse genetic and environmental risk factors for schizophrenia, it seems possible or even probable that schizophrenia is the final common pathway for more than one different neuropathological mechanism, which may have different effects on cognitive impairment. My data cannot address this question.

Social explanations

Social explanations would suggest that school performance here is acting as a proxy for social factors such as economic deprivation, poor housing or lack of social capital. If poor school performance were merely acting as a marker for such social factors, one would expect the effect to be modulated to some extent by social covariates, such as socioeconomic group, migrant status or parental education. However, adding these social variables did not change the association between school grades and schizophrenia. Furthermore, as I have outlined on page 7, it is likely that social risk factors may themselves act via more proximate cognitive or biological mechanisms.

Psychological explanations

Psychological explanations would postulate that poor school performance is a marker for some cognitive deficit, which directly increases risk for schizophrenia. There is a very large literature on cognitive theories of schizophrenia. Anthony David and others have proposed that people with low intelligence may be more prone to make delusional inferences because they are less adept at weighing up the evidence for and against rational versus delusional interpretations of their experiences (David et al., 1997). Philippa Garety, Emmanuelle Peters and colleagues have demonstrated a tendency for schizophrenic patients to jump to conclusions on the basis of flimsy evidence (Peters et al., 2008). Chris Frith has suggested that hallucinations may arise as a consequence of impaired self-monitoring (Frith & Done, 1989). Jenny Barnett and colleagues have recast some of these theories in terms of a protective effect of cognitive reserve, which not only reduces risk for schizophrenia but also improves the outcomes of those affected (Barnett et al., 2006). My data are compatible with explanations of this type.

Intelligence, and other, more specific cognitive phenotypes, are substantially heritable quantitative traits, and any population will contain individuals with poor cognitive functioning. It may be that individuals who happen to be near the lower end of the performance spectrum are at enhanced risk of psychosis because of their psychological deficits, and no further explanation is needed. However, psychological models such as these are perfectly compatible with the view that cognitive deficits in schizophrenia result from neurodevelopmental impairment. If this were the case, cognitive deficits would be best conceptualised as being on the causal pathway between neurodevelopmental impairment and schizophrenia. Note that this differs from the biological model described in on page 133, in which cognitive deficits are merely indicators of neurodevelopmental deviance, and it is the neurodevelopmental deviance itself that predisposes to psychosis.

My conclusion, therefore, is that biological or psychological mechanisms, or a combination of both, are more likely explanations for the association between school performance and schizophrenia than social factors. This does not imply, of course, that social factors are not important in the aetiology of schizophrenia.

The association between school performance and schizoaffective disorder

The most striking finding with regard to schizoaffective disorder is that the association is of the same magnitude and pattern as for schizophrenia, but completely different to that of bipolar disorder. All the same arguments apply as for schizophrenia, and it seems very likely that the same mechanisms underlie both disorders.

The association between school performance and bipolar disorder

U-shaped associations are common in epidemiology. For example, body mass index (Song et al., 2007), hours of sleep (Knutson & Turek, 2006) and alcohol consumption (Imhof et al., 2001) all have U-shaped or J-shaped associations with mortality.

There are two general types of explanation for such associations. The first type of explanation is that there is an ideal value, and any deviation from it increases risk, regardless of direction. For example, there is an ideal curvature for the cornea that will focus light on the retina, and deviations in either direction will degrade visual acuity (expressed in terms of risk, it will increase the risk of requiring spectacles). The second type of explanation is that the U-shaped association results from a combination of two different mechanisms, one of which increases risk at lower levels of the exposure, and the other of which increases risk at higher levels. For example, very low body mass index is associated with advanced neoplastic disease, whereas very high body mass index is associated with cardiovascular disease: the combination of these associations produces a U-shaped association between body mass index and mortality in the population.

The first type of explanation could conceivably explain the relationship between school performance and bipolar disorder, if, for example, performing at an average level was associated with good social functioning, whereas being at either extreme of school performance, regardless of whether high or low, was associated with social isolation. However, I consider it more likely that there are two separate effects operating in bipolar – an effect of low school grades and another effect of high grades, and/or high parental education or socioeconomic group. It might be helpful to conceptualise bipolar disorder as consisting of two different subgroups with different aetiologies – one associated with low, and the other with high school grades.

Poor school performance and bipolar disorder

The arguments that I have advanced above to explain the association between poor school performance in schizophrenia apply equally to bipolar. Given the genetic overlap between the disorders, it may be that the subgroup of bipolar patients who have poor cognitive functioning has similar aetiology as schizophrenia.

Excellent school performance and bipolar disorder

Before considering the putative mechanisms for this association, it is important to note that this association is not nearly as robust as the association between poor school performance and schizophrenia. First, the association seems to be confined to individuals with school performance in the exceptionally gifted range, over 2 standard deviations above the mean, a category that contains the top 1.3% of the population. Second, it seems to be stronger in males than in females. Third, it does not occur in all school subjects. Indeed, high scores in sports and handicrafts seem to be moderately protective against bipolar. Fourth, this is a novel finding that has not been replicated in published studies.

As with schizophrenia, we can focus our thinking by systematically categorising possible explanations. I have discussed the possibilities of chance, bias, reverse causality and confounding, and a direct causal effect of school performance on risk of disease is as unlikely in bipolar disorder as it is in schizophrenia. We are therefore left with the same three categories of indirect association as we were for schizophrenia: biological, social or psychological.

Biological

There is much less evidence of neurodevelopmental impairment or biological environmental risk factors in bipolar disorder than in schizophrenia. Biological mechanisms will therefore be more likely to involve inherited characteristics that both enhance cognitive function, and induce bipolar disorder as a secondary effect. But how might genes predispose to disease and simultaneously to high cognitive functioning?

In a large, stable population, the prevalence of alleles that predispose to disease will tend to decrease to zero given sufficient evolutionary time (Griffiths et al., 1993). However, in some circumstances, the disease-causing allele may have a selective advantage, leading to a balanced polymorphism. The most studied type of balanced polymorphism is heterozygote advantage. In a well-known example of this phenomenon, homozygotes for a mutant allele of the gene coding for the beta polypeptide of the haemoglobin molecule inevitably develop sickle cell anaemia, but heterozygotes are at a selective advantage compared with those with no risk alleles, since heterozygosity confers resistance against malaria. Because of the relative abundance of heterozygotes compared with homozygotes, this survival advantage among heterozygotes counterbalances the much larger disadvantage in homozygotes, and the allele frequency is maintained at around 10%, giving around 1% prevalence of sickle cell disease (Gardner et al., 1991).

The simple model of heterozygote advantage described above was originally applied to single gene disorders, but it could apply to one or more of the genes predisposing to bipolar disorder. For example, heterozygotes, with one risk allele for bipolar, might have enhanced cognitive abilities in a particular domain, whereas homozygotes would have very good cognitive function in that domain but be at increased risk of bipolar disorder.

A more recent model for understanding balanced polymorphisms in multiple genes simultaneously is the concept of stabilising selection. Many continuous, polygenic phenotypes, such as birthweight or anxiety, are normally distributed, with the population mean close to the ideal value of the trait in terms of selective advantage. Stabilising selection is the evolutionary mechanism that is thought to lead to this distribution. At each locus there will be one allele that tends to increase the value of the phenotype, and another which tends to reduce it. Since fitness is generally greatest around the median value of the phenotype, the most adaptive allele at a given locus in a given individual will depend on the genotypes at the other loci. At the population level, therefore, there is no selection pressure favouring one allele at the expense of the other (Walsh, 2003).

For example, consider a hypothetical set of ten genes that control emotional lability, a trait that is normally distributed in the population. At each locus, there is one allele that increases, and another that decreases, emotional lability. The ideal value for emotional lability is intermediate: people whose emotions are very labile are at risk of bipolar disorder and those whose emotions are too flat may have difficulty motivating themselves and perform poorly at emotional activities. At the population level, there is therefore no selection pressure to favour one or other allele at each locus, so the ten polymorphisms will be maintained in the population. People with high levels of emotional lability will be skilled at certain tasks, for example in creative pursuits such as music, but will be at increased risk of bipolar disorder.

Explanations of this type could explain the association between bipolar disorder and excellent school performance, and would also predict that the relatives of bipolar patients would also have high cognitive function. The Icelandic studies of Karlsson (2004) provide some evidence this is the case, although the diagnoses are open to some doubt in these studies (see page 22). The well-replicated finding of higher socioeconomic status in bipolar families (reviewed on page 13) might also be explained by higher cognitive ability in these families.

Social

High parental education was associated with bipolar disorder, and adjusting for parental education attenuated the association between high grades and bipolar. High parental education could be the true risk factor for bipolar disorder, perhaps because highly educated parents drive their children to work harder, leading to mania. Alternatively, it may be that higher parental education simply reflects higher cognitive functioning in relatives, as discussed above.

Psychological

Hypomania is also associated with apparently enhanced access to vocabulary, memory and other cognitive resources. The thought disorder associated with bipolar disorder is characterised by flight of ideas, in which successive thoughts are linked in innovative ways, and patients in this mental state can often be witty, inventive and sharp. It is not difficult to see how these cognitive traits could be associated with good school performance. An unusually strong experience of, or response to, emotional states could also be associated with both affective symptoms and some artistic or creative abilities, as discussed on page 136.

If creativity is indeed associated with bipolar disorder, then one might expect the creative school subjects to be most strongly associated with bipolar disorder. Creativity is not consistently defined, but of the compulsory school subjects taught in Sweden, art, music and Swedish (which includes creative writing) seem intuitively to be closest to the concept of creativity. It is notable that high scores in Swedish and music are risk factors for bipolar disorder, although the association with art is less strong.

There is some anecdotal evidence that the creative output of some individuals with bipolar disorder coincides with periods of mania. In a study on 47 eminent British writers and artists, Kay Redfield Jamison asked respondents about mood disorders and their relationship to periods of productivity. Around one-third had received drug treatment or been hospitalised for mood disorders, and almost all (89%) described intense, highly productive creative periods, characterised by elevated mood and energy, decreased need for sleep, rapid associations between ideas and many other features that resembled hypomanic mental states. The vast majority saw these episodes as very important or essential to their creative output (Jamison, 1989).

The relationship between bipolar disorder and schizophrenia

In the first chapter, I discussed the similarities and differences between bipolar disorder and schizophrenia. My data add to the evidence that schizophrenia and bipolar disorder have very different cognitive profiles, suggesting important differences in aetiology. Schizoaffective disorder seems to have the same pattern of pre-morbid functioning as schizophrenia.

One explanation for the difference in pre-morbid cognitive function between schizophrenia and bipolar disorder is that some or all cases of schizophrenia are a result of neurodevelopmental impairment (reflected in poor school performance), but that patients with bipolar disorder are neurodevelopmentally normal (Demjaha et al., in press). It may also be that there are two biologically distinct disorders, one associated with neurodevelopment and the other not, but that these do not map exactly onto the clinical phenotypes of bipolar and schizophrenia. In other words, 'neurodevelopmental' cases will usually, but not always, have predominantly schizophrenia-like symptoms but may occasionally also show mood symptoms. Non-neurodevelopmental cases will tend to show mainly affective symptoms, but may also suffer from psychotic symptoms.

Perhaps the most parsimonious model, taking into account our knowledge of the genetic and environmental aetiology of both disorders, is that common genetic or environmental risk factors predispose an individual to develop any psychotic disorder, but that these factors alone are often insufficient to cause disease. Psychosis will only occur in those with additional risk factors: those with a neurodevelopmental insult, prolonged stress in childhood or excessive cannabis consumption in adolescence will tend to suffer psychotic symptoms, whereas those with extreme values of particular cognitive or emotional traits will experience bipolar disorder, particularly following life events that give rise to extremes of emotion.

CLINICAL IMPLICATIONS

Utility of school grades in clinical settings

Most previous studies on pre-morbid cognitive function in psychosis have used scores from cognitive tests. These tests may have better reliability than school grades, but most children do not undergo such testing, and if they do, are often not aware of the results.

School performance has an important advantage in this respect. Almost everyone knows his school grades, or at least has some knowledge of how he performed in comparison to his peers. School performance is often incorporated into routine psychiatric assessments (Goldberg & Murray, 2006), and the knowledge that school performance is associated with risk for psychosis is therefore of some clinical utility. In a patient with apparent prodromal symptoms, and/or a high genetic risk for psychosis, poor school performance or a history of missing examinations or assessments this might increase the suspicion of a psychotic disorder. Similarly, very high performance may indicate that the problem is more likely to be bipolar disorder than schizophrenia or schizoaffective disorder.

Prediction or prevention of psychosis at the population level

A hypothetical intervention that was 100% effective in preventing all schizophrenia cases in the population attributable to being in the two lowest school performance categories would eliminate about 17% of cases of schizophrenia (population attributable fractions for lowest and second-lowest categories are 7.4% and 9.7%). If achievable, this would clearly be a worthwhile reduction.

However, the main barrier to prevention is that poor school performance is probably not a preventable risk factor in the way that, for example, smoking is a preventable risk factor for lung cancer. It is difficult to envisage a public health intervention that would improve overall school performance that is not already in place; the very purpose of education systems is to maximise the academic potential of their pupils. Even assuming that such an intervention were available, it would only be effective if poor educational functioning directly influenced risk for psychosis. But as I have argued above, it seems more likely that poor school performance is not a direct cause of psychosis, but a proxy for below-average cognitive function, motivation, behaviour, social skills or some combination of these. If this is correct, then increasing the performance of the entire population will have no effect on the incidence rate of psychosis, since relative performance is merely acting as an indicator of some underlying abnormality, and in any case, it is relative rather than absolute performance that is predictive of psychosis.

If school performance probably cannot be improved, and if this would not prevent psychosis even if it were possible, then is there another intervention that could be used in children who fall into high-risk groups? Clearly, administering any mental health intervention would be ethically questionable in asymptomatic adolescents, who may be too young to give informed consent, and may be stigmatised by the intervention. Moreover, there is no intervention of proven benefit in the primary prevention of psychosis.

The interventions with the best evidence for secondary prevention (i.e. after prodromal symptoms have been detected) are cognitive–behavioural therapy (CBT) and antipsychotic drugs (Lee et al., 2005). Might these approaches be helpful in primary prevention? CBT focuses on the re-interpretation and/or distraction from psychotic symptoms, so it would be of doubtful efficacy in people who have no symptoms. Antipsychotic drugs given at an early stage have arguably shown some promise in secondary prevention, but the ethical implications of prescribing psychotropic drugs for large numbers of healthy adolescents make this approach even less acceptable than psychological approaches.

REMAINING QUESTIONS AND FUTURE DIRECTIONS

It is clear that schizophrenia is associated with pre-morbid cognitive deficits, and this study has shown that these are detectable via school grades, whereas previous Finnish studies did not. Further replications using educational data would help to clarify whether school performance is a predictor of psychosis in other countries. Similarly, our findings in bipolar disorder would be strengthened by replication.

There are three further issues that I aim to explore in the near future, using this and similar data. First, I have information on sibships in the dataset. This will enable me to calculate each individual's family mean GPA and his own deviance from the family mean. This will clarify whether the association between poor school performance and risk for psychosis is operating at the between-family level or the individual level within families. If the effect is mainly at the family level, meaning that being from a family that does poorly at school is the true risk factor, regardless of one's own performance, then factors that pertain to all members of a family are likely to be involved – shared environmental effects such as social status, and some genetic factors. Conversely, if performing worse than one's siblings is a stronger predictor, then individual-level characteristics, for example neurodevelopmental deviance or the psychological consequences of performing worse than one's siblings, are more likely to be important.

The second issue relates to the timing of deficits. I am making plans to obtain access to a new dataset, which includes school grades at age 12–13 and 15–16 for a subsample of the population, and also grades at age 18 for the approximately 75% of individuals who apply to undertake further education in Sweden. These three time-points will allow me to monitor the trajectory of any decline in school performance through childhood.

The third issue is that of the relationship between school performance and cognitive tests. In the subsample described above, there are cognitive test data at age 12–13 for all individuals, and at around 18 years for males only (conscription data). I should be able to determine whether the results of cognitive tests or school performance are stronger predictors of psychosis, and whether psychosis is associated with any particular pattern of discrepancies between cognitive tests and school performance.

The final issue is the impact of family history on the relationship between cognitive function and psychosis. In the new dataset described above, I will have information from the Hospital Discharge Register on diagnoses of psychotic disorders in the parents, allowing me to explore confounding and interaction with familial risk of schizophrenia.

CONCLUSIONS

Poor school performance is a risk factor for schizophrenia and schizoaffective disorder, but only weakly associated with bipolar disorder. Excellent school performance is a risk factor for bipolar disorder. These associations are not confounded by the social and biological factors that I was able to measure. These results indicate a clear discontinuity between schizophrenia and bipolar disorder, and suggest that schizophrenia is associated with neurodevelopmental impairment, whereas bipolar disorder is not. These findings are likely to be of some use in clinical settings but are unlikely to lead to any successful public health interventions.

Appendix

MODEL FITTING FOR SCHIZOPHRENIA

Model 1: unadjusted

Model 1 was the unadjusted Poisson regression model which was presented in Table 5.9 and is repeated as Table A.1 for clarity.

TABLE A.1
Model 1: hazard ratios for schizophrenia, unadjusted

GPA Z-score	Hazard ratio	p>z	95% confidence interval
Below −2	4.08	<0.001	2.99 to 5.56
−2 to −1	1.97	<0.001	1.57 to 2.46
−1 to +1 (ref)	1.00	–	– –
+1 to +2	0.88	0.415	0.65 to 1.20
Over +2	0.00	0.985	– –

Model 2: interaction with age

I tested for an interaction with age (on exit from the study). It should be noted that age does not satisfy the requirements of a potential confounder, as it is not associated with the exposure or outcome. In other words, age at study exit is unrelated to grade-point average (mean GPA for exited study at age <20=3.24; at age 20–25=3.24; at age >25=3.22) and is also only moderately related to risk for schizophrenia (Table 6.1).

As expected, age was not a confounder: adding age band as expanded indicator variables did not change any of the hazard ratios for GPA Z-score by more than 0.01, so all hazard ratios were exactly as in Table A.1. I then compared this with a fully interacting model (Table A.2), using a likelihood ratio test. There was no evidence of interaction with age (likelihood ratio (LR) $\chi^2(8df)=5.57$, p=0.70), so I dropped age from the model.

TABLE A.2
Model 2: interaction between age and grade-point average (GPA) Z-score

Parameter	Hazard ratio	p>z	95% confidence interval
GPA Z-score			
Below –2	3.06	<0.001	1.63 to 5.72
–2 to –1	2.18	<0.001	1.48 to 3.20
–1 to +1 (ref)	1.00	–	– –
+1 to +2	0.68	0.214	0.37 to 1.25
Over +2	0.00	0.990	– –
Age			
Age 20–25	1.17	0.245	0.90 to 1.52
Age >25	0.61	0.012	0.42 to 0.90
GPA × Age			
GPA <–2 × Age 20–25	1.60	0.213	0.76 to 3.33
GPA <–2 × Age >25	1.05	0.932	0.34 to 3.23
GPA –2 to –1 × Age 20–25	0.87	0.576	0.53 to 1.42
GPA –2 to –1 × Age >25	0.83	0.632	0.40 to 1.75
GPA +2 to +1 × Age 20–25	1.26	0.532	0.61 to 2.63
GPA +2 to +1 × Age >25	2.11	0.113	0.84 to 5.30
GPA >2 × Age 20–25	0.86	1.000	– –
GPA >2 × Age >25	1.63	1.000	– –

Model 3: adjusted for sex

Since sex was strongly associated with both school performance and risk for schizophrenia, it seemed the most likely confounder. I had already shown that males were more likely to get schizophrenia, and gained lower marks at school than females; could the association between low school marks and schizophrenia be explained away by adding sex into the model? The answer was no, although adjusting for sex did slightly diminish the strength of the association (Table A.3).

TABLE A.3
Model 3: hazard ratios for schizophrenia, adjusted for sex (female
sex is the exposure group, male sex is the reference group)

GPA Z-score	Hazard ratio	p>z	95% confidence interval
Below −2	3.71	<0.001	2.72 to 5.07
−2 to −1	1.82	<0.001	1.45 to 2.29
−1 to +1 (ref)	1.00	−	− −
+1 to +2	0.95	0.721	0.70 to 1.29
Over +2	0.00	0.983	− −
Female	0.60	<0.001	0.50 to 0.73

GPA, grade-point average.

Model 4: interaction with sex

I then performed an analysis stratified on sex, to look for any suggestion of a different relationship between school performance and schizophrenia in males and females (interaction) (Tables A.4 and A.5).

TABLE A.4
Males

GPA Z-score	Hazard ratio	p>z	95% confidence interval
Below −2	3.19	<0.001	2.22 to 4.60
−2 to −1	1.65	<0.001	1.26 to 2.15
−1 to +1 (ref)	1.00	−	− −
+1 to +2	0.84	0.428	0.54 to 1.30
Over +2	0.00	0.986	− −

GPA, grade-point average.

TABLE A.5
Females

GPA Z-score	Hazard ratio	p>z	95% confidence interval
Below −2	5.63	<0.001	3.15 to 10.06
−2 to −1	2.32	<0.001	1.52 to 3.55
−1 to +1 (ref)	1.00	−	− −
+1 to +2	1.11	0.644	0.72 to 1.71
Over +2	0.00	0.982	− −

GPA, grade-point average.

At first sight, there is a suggestion of a stronger relationship between school performance and schizophrenia in females than males. However, this impression may be misleading, since the distribution of scores is shifted to the right in females compared with males (see Figure 5.3). The Z-score cut-offs were calculated using combined data from both sexes, rather than individually by sex. Therefore, the 'below -2' category represents a more extreme group for females than for males. 3.95% of males in the population fell into that category, but only 1.71% of females (see Table 5.2).

I formally tested for an interaction with sex, by fitting model 4 (not shown) that included interaction terms between sex and every level of school performance, and comparing this with model 2 using a likelihood ratio test. This was not significant, indicating no interaction with sex (LR $\chi^2(4df)=3.91$, p=0.42).

Model 5: adjusted for sex and socioeconomic group.

Socioeconomic group was also strongly associated with both school performance and schizophrenia, so I added this next. I first tested for departure from a linear trend by comparing a model with a linear term for socio-economic group to a fully specified model, using a likelihood ratio test. The fully-specified model was a significantly better fit (LR $\chi^2(4df)=12.5$, p=0.014) (Table A.6). As can be seen in Table A.6, there has been a small

TABLE A.6
Model 5: hazard ratios for schizophrenia, adjusted for sex and socioeconomic group (SEG)

Parameter	Hazard ratio	p>z	95% confidence interval
GPA Z-score			
Below -2	3.62	<0.001	2.62 to 5.00
-2 to -1	1.74	<0.001	1.37 to 2.20
-1 to $+1$ (ref)	1.00	–	– –
$+1$ to $+2$	0.94	0.700	0.69 to 1.29
Over $+2$	0.00	0.982	– –
Female	0.58	<0.001	0.48 to 0.71
SEG			
SEG 1	1.52	0.011	1.10 to 2.11
SEG 2	1.15	0.359	0.85 to 1.56
SEG 3	0.96	0.807	0.69 to 1.34
SEG 5	1.34	0.042	1.01 to 1.77
SEG 6	0.83	0.266	0.61 to 1.15

GPA, grade-point average.

change in the hazard ratios for school performance, where the effect of very low performance has weakened somewhat.

Model 6: adjusted for sex, socioeconomic status and family size

Family size had modest associations with both schizophrenia risk and GPA, so I added this next, as a simple indicator variable for Family size >1. The parameters for this model are shown in Table A.7.

TABLE A.7
Model 6: hazard ratios for schizophrenia, adjusted for sex, socioeconomic group (SEG) and family size

Parameter	Hazard ratio	$p > z$	95% confidence interval
GPA Z-score			
−2	3.54	<0.001	2.56 to 4.89
−2 to −1	1.71	<0.001	1.35 to 2.17
−1 to +1 (ref)	1.00	−	− −
+1 to +2	0.95	0.755	0.70 to 1.30
Over +2	0.00	0.975	− −
Female	0.58	<0.001	0.47 to 0.70
Socioeconomic group (SEG)			
SEG 1	1.51	0.012	1.09 to 2.09
SEG 2	1.15	0.354	0.85 to 1.56
SEG 3	0.95	0.765	0.68 to 1.33
SEG 5	1.34	0.039	1.01 to 1.78
SEG 6	0.83	0.261	0.60 to 1.15
Family size>1	1.24	0.021	1.03 to 1.49

GPA, grade-point average.

Again, there was a small reduction in the strength of association between GPA and risk for schizophrenia.

Model 7: adjusted for sex, socioeconomic status, family size and parental education

I reasoned that the next most likely confounder would be parental education. This was strongly associated with school performance (Figure 6.2), and had a U-shaped association with schizophrenia. It was therefore illogical to add it as a linear term, and I used indicator variables instead. The results are presented in Table A.8.

Adding parental education had two effects. First, there was no evidence that parental education was confounding the association between school

TABLE A.8
Model 7: hazard ratios for schizophrenia, adjusted for sex,
socioeconomic group (SEG), family size and parental education

Parameter	Hazard ratio	$p>z$	95% confidence interval
GPA Z-score			
−2	3.83	<0.001	2.76 to 5.31
−2 to −1	1.84	<0.001	1.44 to 2.34
−1 to +1 (ref)	1.00	–	– –
+1 to +2	0.86	0.341	0.63 to 1.18
Over +2	0.00	0.980	– –
Female	0.59	<0.001	0.48 to 0.72
Socioeconomic group (SEG)			
SEG 1	1.94	<0.001	1.36 to 2.76
SEG 2	1.43	0.035	1.02 to 1.98
SEG 3	1.17	0.397	0.82 to 1.66
SEG 5	1.06	0.720	0.79 to 1.42
SEG 6	0.93	0.645	0.67 to 1.28
Family size>1	1.30	0.006	1.08 to 1.56
Parental education			
Parental education 1	0.87	0.470	0.59 to 1.28
Parental education 2	1.00	0.992	0.73 to 1.37
Parental education 4	1.20	0.329	0.83 to 1.73
Parental education 5	2.10	<0.001	1.50 to 2.95

GPA, grade-point average.

performance and schizophrenia. Indeed, adding parental education to the model actually strengthened the association between GPA and schizophrenia risk.

Second, parental education, now that it was adjusted for socioeconomic group, GPA and the other confounders, seemed to have a linear association with schizophrenia risk, such that individuals whose parents had higher levels of education had greater risks of schizophrenia. This suggested that perhaps there was an interaction between parental education and school performance (poor school performance may have been a stronger risk factor in people with highly educated parents).

Model 8: adjusted for sex, socioeconomic status and family size, with an interaction between grade-point average and parental education

I tested for an interaction between school performance and parental education by specifying a model which included interaction terms between each of the indicator variables for GPA with each of the indicator variables for parental education. I compared the resulting model 8 (not shown) with model 7, using a likelihood ratio test, and found no evidence that model 8 was a better fit than model 7 (LR $\chi^2(16df)=16.1$, p=0.449).

MODEL FITTING FOR SCHIZOAFFECTIVE DISORDER

Model 1: unadjusted

Model 1 was the unadjusted Poisson regression model which was presented in Table 5.1, and is repeated as Table A.9 for clarity.

TABLE A.9
Model 1: hazard ratios for schizoaffective disorder, unadjusted

GPA Z-score	Hazard ratio	p>z	95% confidence interval
Below −2	3.81	<0.001	1.81 to 8.03
−2 to −1	2.70	<0.001	1.68 to 4.33
−1 to +1 (ref)	1.00	–	– –
+1 to +2	0.71	0.386	0.32 to 1.55
Over +2	0.00	0.982	– –

GPA, grade-point average.

Model 2: interaction with age

Model 2 included interaction terms for age (Table A.10). Comparing this with a model including age but no interactions (in which the hazard ratios for school performance were almost identical to model 1, so not shown), there was no evidence of interaction with age (LR $\chi^2(8df)=6.89$, p=0.55), so I dropped age from the model.

Model 3: interaction with sex

The relationship between school performance and schizoaffective disorder is stronger in males (Table A.11) than females (Table A.12). However, a likelihood ratio test showed no evidence of interaction with sex (LR $\chi^2(4df)=3.97$, p=0.41), so this model was also rejected.

TABLE A.10
Model 2: hazard ratios for schizoaffective disorder, with
interaction terms for age

Parameter	Hazard ratio	p>z	95% confidence interval
GPA Z-score			
Below −2	4.37	0.019	1.28 to 14.90
−2 to −1	2.53	0.030	1.09 to 5.86
−1 to +1 (ref)	1.00	–	– –
+1 to +2	1.49	0.434	0.55 to 4.04
Over +2	0.00	0.996	– –
Age			
Age 20–25	1.11	0.732	0.61 to 2.03
Age >25	0.52	0.168	0.20 to 1.32
GPA × age			
GPA <−2 × Age 20–25	0.99	0.991	0.21 to 4.69
GPA <−2 × Age >25	0.00	0.994	– –
GPA −2 to −1 × Age 20–25	1.04	0.935	0.36 to 3.01
GPA −2 to −1 × Age >25	1.36	0.691	0.30 to 6.22
GPA +2 to +1 × Age 20–25	0.24	0.115	0.04 to 1.41
GPA +2 to +1 × Age >25	0.00	0.989	– –
GPA >2 × Age 20–25	0.90	1.000	– –
GPA >2 × Age >25	1.92	1.000	– –

GPA, grade-point average.

TABLE A.11
Males

GPA Z-score	Hazard ratio	p>z	95% confidence interval
Below −2	4.53	<0.001	0.000 to 1.97
−2 to −1	2.24	<0.001	0.012 to 1.19
−1 to +1 (ref)	1.00	–	– –
+1 to +2	0.26	0.188	0.04 to 1.93
Over +2	0.00	0.987	– –

GPA, grade-point average.

TABLE A.12
Females

GPA Z-score	Hazard ratio	p>z	95% confidence interval
Below −2	1.70	0.605	0.23 to 12.54
−2 to −1	3.58	0.000	1.75 to 7.30
−1 to +1 (ref)	1.00	–	– –
+1 to +2	1.00	0.998	0.41 to 2.45
Over +2	0.00	0.985	– –

GPA, grade-point average.

Model 4: adjusted for preterm delivery

Adjusting for preterm delivery slightly attenuated the association between school performance and schizoaffective disorder, suggesting that preterm delivery may have been acting as a confounder (Table A.13, compare with Table A.9).

TABLE A.13
Hazard ratios for schizoaffective disorder, adjusted for preterm delivery

Parameter	Hazard ratio	p>z	95% confidence interval
GPA Z-score			
Below −2	3.77	0.000	1.79 to 7.95
−2 to −1	2.68	0.000	1.67 to 4.30
−1 to +1 (ref)	1.00	–	– –
+1 to +2	0.71	0.391	0.32 to 1.56
Over +2	0.00	0.986	– –
Preterm delivery	1.81	0.158	0.79 to 4.15

GPA, grade-point average.

Model 5: adjusted for preterm delivery and birth order

As predicted, adjusting for birth order reveals a modest degree of negative confounding: the association between school performance and schizoaffective disorder becomes somewhat stronger after controlling for birth order (Table A.14).

TABLE A.14
Hazard ratios for schizoaffective disorder, adjusted for preterm delivery and birth order

Parameter	Hazard ratio	p>z	95% confidence interval
GPA Z-score			
Below −2	3.99	0.000	1.89 to 8.43
−2 to −1	2.77	0.000	1.73 to 4.45
−1 to +1 (ref)	1.00	–	– –
+1 to +2	0.69	0.354	0.31 to 1.52
Over +2	0.00	0.982	– –
Preterm delivery	1.82	0.158	0.79 to 4.16
Birth order			
Second born	0.73	0.159	0.46 to 1.13
Third born or greater	0.50	0.033	0.27 to 0.94

GPA, grade-point average.

MODEL FITTING FOR BIPOLAR DISORDER

Model 1: unadjusted

Model 1 was the unadjusted Poisson regression model that was presented in Table 5.11, and is repeated as Table A.15 for clarity.

TABLE A.15
Model 1: hazard ratios for bipolar disorder, unadjusted

GPA Z-score	Hazard ratio	p>z	95% confidence interval
Below −2	1.89	0.027	1.08 to 3.33
−2 to −1	1.20	0.302	0.85 to 1.71
−1 to +1 (ref)	1.00	–	– –
+1 to +2	1.48	0.017	1.07 to 2.04
Over +2	3.52	<0.001	1.86 to 6.66

GPA, grade-point average.

Model 2: interaction with age

As with schizophrenia, I tested for an interaction with age by comparing a model including age (in which the hazard ratios for school performance were almost identical to model 1) with a fully interacting model (Table A.16), using a likelihood ratio test. There was no evidence of interaction with age (LR χ^2(8df)=11.98, p=0.15), so I dropped age from the model.

Model 3: interaction with sex

Table A.17 (males) and Table A.18 (females) show the results stratified by sex. The association of high school performance with bipolar disorder is much stronger in males than females.

The association between poor school performance and bipolar seems to be confined to females. However, the distributions of males and females in the various school performance categories, differ markedly by sex, with females outperforming males (see Figure 5.3 and Table 5.2). It follows that males in the +2 category are a more extreme group than females in the same category, since it is rarer for males to achieve this level of performance than females. Similarly, females in the −2 category are probably more impaired than males in that category.

Since bipolar disorder seems to affect both males and females approximately equally, we would not expect sex to confound the association

TABLE A.16
Model 2: hazard ratios for bipolar disorder, with interaction
terms for age

Parameter	Hazard ratio	p>z	95% confidence interval
GPA Z-score			
Below −2	1.67	0.266	0.68 to 4.14
−2 to −1	1.53	0.087	0.94 to 2.48
−1 to +1 (ref)	1.00	–	– –
+1 to +2	1.57	0.058	0.99 to 2.51
Over +2	6.14	<0.001	2.96 to 12.73
Age			
Age 20–25	0.69	0.025	0.50 to 0.95
Age >25	0.34	<0.001	0.20 to 0.57
GPA × Age			
GPA <−2 × Age 20–25	1.53	0.476	0.48 to 4.88
GPA <−2 × Age >25	0.00	0.984	– –
GPA −2 to −1 × Age 20–25	0.64	0.240	0.30 to 1.35
GPA −2 to −1 × Age >25	0.60	0.444	0.16 to 2.24
GPA +2 to +1 × Age 20–25	0.77	0.458	0.38 to 1.54
GPA +2 to +1 × Age >25	1.39	0.514	0.51 to 3.78
GPA >2 × Age 20–25	0.25	0.085	0.05 to 1.21
GPA >2 × Age >25	0.00	0.989	– –

GPA, grade-point average.

TABLE A.17
Males

GPA Z-score	Hazard ratio	p>z	95% confidence interval
Below −2	1.53	0.281	0.71 to 3.31
−2 to −1	0.91	0.709	0.54 to 1.51
−1 to +1 (ref)	1.00	–	– –
+1 to +2	1.59	0.075	0.95 to 2.65
Over +2	6.62	<0.001	2.68 to 16.34

GPA, grade-point average.

TABLE A.18
Females

GPA Z-score	Hazard ratio	p>z	95% confidence interval
Below −2	2.81	0.014	1.23 to 6.42
−2 to −1	1.79	0.018	1.10 to 2.92
−1 to +1 (ref)	1.00	–	– –
+1 to +2	1.38	0.127	0.91 to 2.09
Over +2	2.31	0.068	0.94 to 5.70

GPA, grade-point average.

between school performance and bipolar disorder. However, adding sex to the model did lead to a small change in some of the hazard ratios, so I have included this model for completeness (Table A.19).

TABLE A.19
Model 3a: hazard ratios for bipolar disorder, controlling for sex

GPA Z-score	Hazard ratio	p>z	95% confidence interval
Below −2	1.96	0.020	1.11 to 3.46
−2 to −1	1.24	0.236	0.87 to 1.77
−1 to +1 (ref)	1.00	−	− −
+1 to +2	1.44	0.027	1.04 to 1.99
Over +2	3.38	<0.001	1.78 to 6.41
Female	1.20	0.144	0.94 to 1.52

GPA, grade-point average.

I then compared Model 3a (Table A.19) with the fully interacting model (Model 3b, Table A.20) to test for any overall effect of interaction with sex. There was only weak interaction, which was not significant at the $p<0.05$ level, so interaction with sex was rejected (LR $\chi^2(4df)=8.13$, $p=0.09$).

TABLE A.20
Model 3b: hazard ratios for bipolar disorder, interaction with sex

Parameter	Hazard ratio	p>z	95% confidence interval
GPA Z-score			
Below −2	1.53	0.281	0.71 to 3.31
−2 to −1	0.91	0.709	0.54 to 1.51
−1 to +1 (ref)	1.00	−	− −
+1 to +2	1.59	0.075	0.95 to 2.65
Over +2	6.62	<0.001	2.68 to 16.34
Female	1.12	0.454	0.83 to 1.52
GPA × Female			
Below −2 × female	1.84	0.293	0.59 to 5.70
−2 to −1 × female	1.98	0.058	0.98 to 4.00
+1 to +2 × female	0.87	0.674	0.45 to 1.68
Over +2 × female	0.35	0.106	0.10 to 1.25

GPA, grade-point average.

Model 4: adjusting for parental education

Adding parental education to the model had some very interesting effects (Table A.21). The association between high school performance and bipolar disorder was attenuated, suggesting that parental education was confounding this relationship. However, the association between low school performance and bipolar disorder was accentuated, suggesting some negative confounding (unmasking of a true effect). In other words, the relationship between high school performance and bipolar may be partly explained by bipolar patients having high parental education, whereas the relationship between low school performance and bipolar was masked by the fact that bipolar patients had better-educated parents, which had 'pulled up' their scores.

TABLE A.21
Model 4: hazard ratios for bipolar disorder, adjusted for parental education

Parameter	Hazard ratio	p>z	95% confidence interval
GPA Z-score			
Below –2	2.19	0.007	1.23 to 3.87
–2 to –1	1.35	0.101	0.94 to 1.94
–1 to +1 (ref)	1.00	–	– –
+1 to +2	1.29	0.131	0.93 to 1.80
Over +2	2.95	0.001	1.55 to 5.65
Parental education			
Parental education 1	0.85	0.543	0.51 to 1.42
Parental education 2	0.92	0.69	0.63 to 1.36
Parental education 4	1.14	0.56	0.74 to 1.75
Parental education 5	1.49	0.043	1.01 to 2.20

GPA, grade-point average.

Model 5: interaction with parental education

Model 4 suggested that there may be a different relationship between GPA and bipolar disorder at different levels of parental education. To test whether there was an interaction, I compared this model 4 with the fully interacting model 5, shown in Table A.22. However, there was no significant interaction (LR χ^2(16df)=20.47, p=0.20).

TABLE A.22
Model 5: hazard ratios for bipolar disorder, interaction with
parental education

Parameter	Hazard ratio	p>z	95% confidence interval
GPA Z-score			
Below −2 (GPA1)	1.61	0.642	0.22 to 11.94
−2 to −1 (GPA2)	1.70	0.248	0.69 to 4.20
−1 to +1 (ref)	1.00	–	– –
+1 to +2 (GPA4)	1.67	0.268	0.68 to 4.11
Over +2 (GPA5)	12.62	<0.001	3.78 to 42.17
Parental education			
Parental education 1 (PE1)	1.11	0.744	0.58 to 2.12
Parental education 2 (PE2)	1.19	0.489	0.73 to 1.96
Parental education 4 (PE4)	1.25	0.424	0.72 to 2.18
Parental education 5 (PE5)	1.53	0.103	0.92 to 2.55
GPA × Parental education	0.83	0.880	0.07 to 9.91
GPA1 × PE1			
GPA1 × PE2	1.29	0.817	0.15 to 11.11
GPA1 × PE4	2.49	0.467	0.21 to 29.30
GPA1 × PE5	1.52	0.772	0.09 to 25.43
GPA2 × PE1	0.74	0.639	0.21 to 2.62
GPA2 × PE2	0.44	0.152	0.15 to 1.35
GPA2 × PE4	0.89	0.865	0.24 to 3.31
GPA2 × PE5	1.91	0.273	0.60 to 6.04
GPA4 × PE1	0.00	0.986	– –
GPA4 × PE2	0.57	0.387	0.16 to 2.05
GPA4 × PE4	0.89	0.851	0.28 to 2.89
GPA4 × PE5	0.89	0.820	0.32 to 2.47
GPA5 × PE1	0.00	0.997	– –
GPA5 × PE2	0.30	0.314	0.03 to 3.08
GPA5 × PE4	0.00	0.991	– –
GPA5 × PE5	0.22	0.046	0.05 to 0.98

GPA, grade-point average.

Model 6: controlling for parental education and preterm delivery

Controlling for preterm delivery resulted in a modest reduction in the association between poor school performance and bipolar disorder (Table A.23, compare with Table A.21).

TABLE A.23
Model 6: hazard ratios for bipolar disorder, controlling for
parental education and preterm delivery

Parameter	Hazard ratio	p>z	95% confidence interval
GPA Z-score			
Below −2	2.16	0.008	1.22 to 3.83
−2 to −1	1.34	0.109	0.94 to 1.92
−1 to +1 (ref)	1.00	–	– –
+1 to +2	1.30	0.125	0.93 to 1.81
Over +2	2.96	0.001	1.55 to 5.66
Parental education			
Parental education 1	0.85	0.526	0.51 to 1.41
Parental education 2	0.92	0.679	0.62 to 1.36
Parental education 4	1.14	0.556	0.74 to 1.75
Parental education 5	1.50	0.041	1.02 to 2.21
Preterm delivery	2.11	0.002	1.33 to 3.37

GPA, grade-point average.

Model 7: controlling for parental education, preterm delivery and head circumference

Controlling for head circumference also modestly reduced the association between low school performance and bipolar disorder (Table A.24).

TABLE A.24
Model 7: hazard ratios for bipolar disorder, controlling for
parental education, preterm delivery and head circumference

Parameter	Hazard ratio	p>z	95% confidence interval
GPA Z-score			
Below −2	2.13	0.010	1.20 to 3.78
−2 to −1	1.33	0.119	0.93 to 1.91
−1 to +1 (ref)	1.00	–	– –
+1 to +2	1.31	0.117	0.94 to 1.82
Over +2	2.98	0.001	1.56 to 5.70
Parental education			
Parental education 1	0.85	0.528	0.51 to 1.41
Parental education 2	0.92	0.680	0.62 to 1.36
Parental education 4	1.14	0.551	0.74 to 1.76
Parental education 5	1.50	0.040	1.02 to 2.21
Preterm delivery	2.10	0.002	1.31 to 3.34
Head circumference			
Low head circumference	1.80	0.027	1.07 to 3.03
High head circumference	0.72	0.517	0.27 to 1.94

GPA, grade-point average.

Model 8: controlling for parental education, preterm delivery, head circumference and advanced paternal age

Adding paternal age >45 to model 7 had almost no effect on the relationship between school performance and bipolar disorder (Table A.25), so model 7 remained the most parsimonious model.

TABLE A.25
Model 8: hazard ratios for bipolar disorder, adjusted for parental education, preterm delivery, head circumference and advanced paternal age

Parameter	Hazard ratio	$p>z$	95% confidence interval
GPA Z-score			
Below −2	2.13	0.010	1.20 to 3.78
−2 to −1	1.33	0.118	0.93 to 1.91
−1 to +1 (ref)	1.00	−	− −
+1 to +2	1.30	0.120	0.93 to 1.82
Over +2	2.97	0.001	1.55 to 5.68
Parental education			
Parental education 1	0.82	0.438	0.49 to 1.36
Parental education 2	0.91	0.655	0.62 to 1.35
Parental education 4	1.14	0.560	0.74 to 1.75
Parental education 5	1.49	0.043	1.01 to 2.20
Preterm delivery	2.09	0.002	1.31 to 3.33
Head circumference			
Low head circumference	1.80	0.027	1.07 to 3.04
High head circumference	0.72	0.507	0.27 to 1.92
Father >45	2.43	0.021	1.14 to 5.17

GPA, grade-point average.

References

Abood, Z., Sharkey, A., Webb, M., Kelly, A., Gill, M. (2002). Are patients with bipolar affective disorder socially disadvantaged? A comparison with a control group. *Bipolar Disorders, 4(4)*, 243–248.

Adityanjee, Aderibigbe, Y.A., Theodoridis, D., Vieweg, V.R. (1999). Dementia praecox to schizophrenia: the first 100 years. *Psychiatry and Clinical Neuroscience, 53(4)*, 437–448.

Agid, O., Shapira, B., Zislin, J., Ritsner, M., Hanin, B., Murad, H., Troudart, T., Bloch, M., Heresco-Levy, U., Lerer, B. (1999). Environment and vulnerability to major psychiatric illness: a case control study of early parental loss in major depression, bipolar disorder and schizophrenia. *Molecular Psychiatry, 4(2)*, 163–172.

American Psychiatric Association (1994). *Diagnostic and statistical manual of mental disorder*, 4th ed. (DSM–IV). Washington: APA.

Andreasen, N.C. (1987). Creativity and mental illness: prevalence rates in writers and their first-degree relatives. *American Journal of Psychiatry, 144(10)*, 1288–1292.

Angst, J., Marneros, A. (2001). Bipolarity from ancient to modern times: conception, birth and rebirth. *Journal of Affective Disorders, 67(1–3)*, 3–19.

Aro, S., Aro, H., Salinto, M., Keskimaki, I. (1995). Educational level and hospital use in mental disorders. A population-based study. *Acta Psychiatrica Scandinavica, 91(5)*, 305–312.

Arvidsson, H., Ericson, B.G. (2005). The development of psychiatric care after the mental health care reform in Sweden. A case register study. *Nordic Journal of Psychiatry, 59(3)*, 186–192.

Barnett, J.H., Salmond, C.H., Jones, P.B., Sahakian, B.J. (2006). Cognitive reserve in neuropsychiatry. *Psychological Medicine, 36(8)*, 1053–1064.

Bebbington, P.E., Bhugra, D., Brugha, T., Singleton, N., Farrell, M., Jenkins, R., Lewis, G., Meltzer, H. (2004). Psychosis, victimisation and childhood disadvantage: evidence from the second British National Survey of Psychiatric Morbidity. *British Journal of Psychiatry, 185*, 220–226.

Bergvall, N., Iliadou, A., Tuvemo, T., Cnattingius, S. (2006). Birth characteristics and risk of low intellectual performance in early adulthood: are the associations confounded by socioeconomic factors in adolescence or familial effects? *Pediatrics*, *117(3)*, 714–721.

Boydell, J., van Os, J., McKenzie, K., Allardyce, J., Goel, R., McCreadie, R.G., Murray, R.M. (2001). Incidence of schizophrenia in ethnic minorities in London: ecological study into interactions with environment. *British Medical Journal*, *323(7325)*, 1336.

Boyer, P., Ramble, C. (2001). Cognitive templates for religious concepts: cross-cultural evidence for recall of counter-intuitive representations. *Cognitive Science*, *25*, 535–564.

Brockington, I.F., Kendell, R.E., Wainwright, S., Hillier, V.F., Walker, J. (1979). The distinction between the affective psychoses and schizophrenia. *British Journal of Psychiatry*, *135*, 243–248.

Brown, A.S. (2006). Prenatal infection as a risk factor for schizophrenia. *Schizophrenia Bulletin*, *32(2)*, 200–202.

Brown, A.S., Begg, M.D., Gravenstein, S., Schaefer, C.A., Wyatt, R.J., Bresnahan, M., Babulas, V.P., Susser, E.S. (2004). Serologic evidence of prenatal influenza in the etiology of schizophrenia. *Archives of General Psychiatry*, *61(8)*, 774–780.

Bundy, H., MacCabe, J.H. (in press). The schizophrenia paradox: a systematic review and meta-analysis of the fertility of schizophrenic patients and their unaffected siblings.

Callas, P.W., Pastides, H., Hosmer, D.W. (1994). Survey of methods and statistical models used in the analysis of occupational cohort studies. *Occupational and Environmental Medicine*, *51(10)*, 649–655.

Callas, P.W., Pastides, H., Hosmer, D.W. (1998). Empirical comparisons of proportional hazards, Poisson, and logistic regression modeling of occupational cohort data. *American Journal of Industrial Medicine*, *33(1)*, 33–47.

Cannon, M., Jones, P., Huttunen, M.O., Tanskanen, A., Huttunen, T., Rabe-Hesketh, S., Murray, R.M. (1999). School performance in Finnish children and later development of schizophrenia: a population-based longitudinal study. *Archives of General Psychiatry*, *56(5)*, 457–463.

Cannon, M., Jones, P.B., Murray, R.M. (2002a). Obstetric complications and schizophrenia: historical and meta-analytic review. *American Journal of Psychiatry*, *159(7)*, 1080–1092.

Cannon, M., Caspi, A., Moffitt, T.E., Harrington, H., Taylor, A., Murray, R.M., Poulton, R. (2002b). Evidence for early-childhood, pan-developmental impairment specific to schizophreniform disorder: results from a longitudinal birth cohort. *Archives of General Psychiatry*, *59(5)*, 449–456.

Cannon, T.D., Bearden, C.E., Hollister, J.M., Rosso, I.M., Sanchez, L.E., Hadley, T. (2000). Childhood cognitive functioning in schizophrenia patients and their unaffected siblings: a prospective cohort study. *Schizophrenia Bulletin*, *26(2)*, 379–393.

Cantor-Graae, E., Selten, J.P. (2005). Schizophrenia and migration: a meta-analysis and review. *American Journal of Psychiatry*, *162(1)*, 12–24.

Cardno, A.G., Marshall, E.J., Coid, B., Macdonald, A.M., Ribchester, T.R., Davies, N.J., Venturi, P., Jones, L.A., Lewis, S.W., Sham, P.C., Gottesman, I.I., Farmer, A.E., McGuffin, P., Reveley, A.M., Murray, R.M. (1999). Heritability estimates for psychotic disorders: the Maudsley twin psychosis series. *Archives of General Psychiatry*, *56(2)*, 162–168.

Cardno, A.G., Rijsdijk, F.V., Sham, P.C., Murray, R.M., McGuffin, P. (2002). A twin study of genetic relationships between psychotic symptoms. *American Journal of Psychiatry*, *159(4)*, 539–545.

Caspi, A., Moffitt, T.E., Cannon, M., McClay, J., Murray, R., Harrington, H., Taylor, A., Arseneault, L., Williams, B., Braithwaite, A., Poulton, R., Craig, I.W. (2005). Moderation of the effect of adolescent-onset cannabis use on adult psychosis by a functional polymorphism in the catechol-O-methyltransferase gene: longitudinal evidence of a gene X environment interaction. *Biological Psychiatry*, *57(10)*, 1117–1127.

Castle, D.J., Scott, K., Wessely, S., Murray, R.M. (1993). Does social deprivation during gestation and early life predispose to later schizophrenia? *Social Psychiatry and Psychiatric Epidemiology*, *28(1)*, 1–4.

Cnattingius, S., Ericson, A., Gunnarskog, J., Kallen, B. (1990). A quality study of a medical birth registry. *Scandinavian Journal of Social Medicine*, *18(2)*, 143–148.

Craddock, N., O'Donovan, M.C., Owen, M.J. (2006). Genes for schizophrenia and bipolar disorder? Implications for psychiatric nosology. *Schizophrenia Bulletin*, *32(1)*, 9–16.

Crow, T.J. (1990). The continuum of psychosis and its genetic origins. The sixty-fifth Maudsley lecture. *British Journal of Psychiatry*, *156*, 788–797.

Curran, C., Byrappa, N., McBride, A. (2004). Stimulant psychosis: systematic review. *British Journal of Psychiatry*, *185*, 196–204.

Dalman, C., Broms, J., Cullberg, J., Allebeck, P. (2002). Young cases of schizophrenia identified in a national inpatient register – are the diagnoses valid? *Social Psychiatry and Psychiatric Epidemiology*, *37(11)*, 527–531.

David, A.S. (1999). Intelligence and schizophrenia. *Acta Psychiatrica Scandinavica*, *100(1)*, 1–2.

David, A.S., Malmberg, A., Brandt, L., Allebeck, P., Lewis, G. (1997). IQ and risk for schizophrenia: a population-based cohort study. *Psychological Medicine*, *27(6)*, 1311–1323.

Davidson, M., Reichenberg, A., Rabinowitz, J., Weiser, M., Kaplan, Z., Mark, M. (1999). Behavioral and intellectual markers for schizophrenia in apparently healthy male adolescents. *American Journal of Psychiatry*, *156(9)*, 1328–1335.

Dean, K., Bramon, E., Murray, R.M. (2003). The causes of schizophrenia: neurodevelopment and other risk factors. *Journal of Psychiatric Practice*, *9(6)*, 442–454.

Deary, I.J. (2001). *Intelligence: a very short introduction*. Oxford: Oxford University Press.

Deary, I.J., Crawford, J.R. (1998). A triarchic theory of Jensenism: persistent, conservative reductionism. *Intelligence*, *26*, 273–282.

Deary, I.J., Strand, P., Smith, P., Fernandes, C. (2007). Intelligence and educational achievement. *Intelligence*, *35(1)*, 13–21.

Demjaha, A., MacCabe, J.H., Murray, R.M. (in press). Schizophrenia and bipolar disorder: the crucial differences are neurodevelopmental. *Annals of Clinical Psychiatry*.

Done, D.J., Crow, T.J., Johnstone, E.C., Sacker, A. (1994). Childhood antecedents of schizophrenia and affective illness: social adjustment at ages 7 and 11. *British Medical Journal*, *309(6956)*, 699–703.

Dryden, J. (2004). *Absalom and Achitophel (Part I)*. Kila, MT: Kessinger Publishing. (Original work published 1681)

Dutta, R., MacCabe, J.H. (in press).

Ekholm, B., Ekholm, A., Adolfsson, R., Vares, M., Osby, U., Sedvall, G.C., Jonsson, E.G. (2005). Evaluation of diagnostic procedures in Swedish patients with schizophrenia and related psychoses. *Nordic Journal of Psychiatry*, *59(6)*, 457–464.

Eysenck, H.J. (1994). The measurement of creativity. In M.A. Boden (ed.), *Dimensions of creativity*. (pp. 199–242). London: The MIT Press.

Fananas, L., Bertranpetit, J. (1995). Reproductive rates in families of schizophrenic patients in a case-control study. *Acta Psychiatrica Scandinavica*, *91(3)*, 202–204.

Farmer, A., Elkin, A., McGuffin, P. (2007). The genetics of bipolar affective disorder. *Current Opinion in Psychiatry*, *20(1)*, 8–12.

Fearon, P., Kirkbride, J.B., Morgan, C., Dazzan, P., Morgan, K., Lloyd, T., Hutchinson, G., Tarrant, J., Fung, W.L., Holloway, J., Mallett, R., Harrison, G., Leff, J., Jones, P.B., Murray, R.M. (2006). Incidence of schizophrenia and other psychoses in ethnic minority groups: results from the MRC AESOP Study. *Psychological Medicine*, *36(11)*, 1541–1550.

Flynn, J.R. (2007). *What is intelligence?* Cambridge: Cambridge University Press.

Frith, C.D., Done, D.J. (1989). Experiences of alien control in schizophrenia reflect a disorder in the central monitoring of action. *Psychological Medicine, 19(2)*, 359–363.

Gardner, E.J., Simmons, M.J., Snustad, D.P. (1991). *Principles of genetics*, 8th ed. Chichester: John Wiley and Sons.

Goldberg, D., Murray, R. (2006). *Maudsley handbook of practical psychiatry*. Oxford: Oxford University Press.

Goleman, D.P. (1995). *Emotional intelligence*. New York: Bantam.

Gonzalez, A. (2003). The education and wages of immigrant children: the impact of age at arrival. *Economics of Education Review, 22(2)*, 203.

Griffiths, A.J.F., Miller, J.H., Suzuki, D.T., Lewontin, R.C., Gelbart, W.M. (1993). *An introduction to genetic analysis*, 5th ed. New York: W.F. Freeman and Co.

Grimes, D.A., Schulz, K.F. (2002). Bias and causal associations in observational research. *Lancet, 359(9302)*, 248–252.

Gunnell, D., Harrison, G., Rasmussen, F., Fouskakis, D., Tynelius, P. (2002). Associations between premorbid intellectual performance, early-life exposures and early-onset schizophrenia. Cohort study. *British Journal of Psychiatry, 181*, 298–305.

Hansson, L. (1989). Utilization of psychiatric inpatient care. A study of changes related to the introduction of a sectorized care organization. *Acta Psychiatrica Scandinavica, 79(6)*, 571–578.

Harrison, G., Gunnell, D., Glazebrook, C., Page, K., Kwiecinski, R. (2001). Association between schizophrenia and social inequality at birth: case-control study. *British Journal of Psychiatry, 179*, 346–350.

Harrison, P.J., Law, A.J. (2006). Neuregulin 1 and schizophrenia: genetics, gene expression, and neurobiology. *Biological Psychiatry, 60(2)*, 132–140.

Heinrichs, R.W., Zakzanis, K.K. (1998). Neurocognitive deficit in schizophrenia: a quantitative review of the evidence. *Neuropsychology, 12(3)*, 426–445.

Henquet, C., Rosa, A., Krabbendam, L., Papiol, S., Fananas, L., Drukker, M., Ramaekers, J.G., van Os, J. (2006a). An experimental study of catechol-o-methyltransferase Val158Met moderation of delta-9-tetrahydrocannabinol-induced effects on psychosis and cognition. *Neuropsychopharmacology, 31(12)*, 2748–2757.

Henquet, C., Krabbendam, L., de Graaf, R., ten Have, M., van Os, J. (2006b). Cannabis use and expression of mania in the general population. *Journal of Affective Disorders, 95(1–3)*, 103–110.

Herrnstein, R.J., Murray, C. (1994). *The bell curve: The reshaping of American life by differences in intelligence*. New York: Free Press.

Hershman, D.J., Lieb, J. (1998). *Manic depression and creativity* (pp. v, 230). Amherst, NY: Prometheus Books.

Higher Education Funding Council of England (HEFCE) (1999). *Performance indicators in higher education in the UK*. Bristol: HEFCE.

Hirschfeld, R.M., Cross, C.K. (1982). Epidemiology of affective disorders. *Archives of General Psychiatry, 39(1)*, 35–46.

Hodgkinson, C.A., Goldman, D., Jaeger, J., Persaud, S., Kane, J.M., Lipsky, R.H., Malhotra, A.K. (2004). Disrupted in schizophrenia 1 (DISC1): association with schizophrenia, schizoaffective disorder, and bipolar disorder. *American Journal of Human Genetics, 75(5)*, 862–872.

Hopper, K., Wanderling, J. (2000). Revisiting the developed versus developing country distinction in course and outcome in schizophrenia: results from ISoS, the WHO collaborative followup project. International Study of Schizophrenia. *Schizophrenia Bulletin, 26(4)*, 835–846.

Hsieh, F.Y., Lavori, P.W. (2000). Sample-size calculations for the Cox proportional hazards regression model with nonbinary covariates. *Controlled Clinical Trials, 21(6)*, 552–560.

Hultman, C.M., Sparen, P., Takei, N., Murray, R.M., Cnattingius, S. (1999). Prenatal and perinatal risk factors for schizophrenia, affective psychosis, and reactive psychosis of early onset: case-control study. *British Medical Journal, 318(7181)*, 421–426.

Imhof, A., Froehlich, M., Brenner, H., Boeing, H., Pepys, M.B., Koenig, W. (2001). Effect of alcohol consumption on systemic markers of inflammation. *Lancet, 357(9258)*, 763–767.

International Schizophrenia Consortium (2008). Rare chromosomal deletions and duplications increase risk of schizophrenia. *Nature, 455(7210)*, 237–241.

Isohanni, I., Jarvelin, M.R., Nieminen, P., Jones, P., Rantakallio, P., Jokelainen, J., Isohanni, M. (1998). School performance as a predictor of psychiatric hospitalization in adult life. A 28-year follow-up in the Northern Finland 1966 Birth Cohort. *Psychological Medicine, 28(4)*, 967–974.

Isohanni, I., Jarvelin, M.R., Jones, P., Jokelainen, J., Isohanni, M. (1999). Can excellent school performance be a precursor of schizophrenia? A 28-year follow-up in the Northern Finland 1966 birth cohort [see comments]. *Acta Psychiatrica Scandinavica, 100(1)*, 17–26.

Jamison, K.R. (1989). Mood disorders and patterns of creativity in British writers and artists. *Psychiatry, 52(2)*, 125–134.

Jamison, K.R. (1993). *Touched with fire: manic depressive illness and the artistic temperament.* New York: Simon & Schuster.

Johnson, S.L. (2005). Life events in bipolar disorder: towards more specific models. *Clinical Psychology Review, 25(8)*, 1008–1027.

Jones, P. (1995). Childhood motor milestones and IQ prior to adult schizophrenia: results from a 43 year old British birth cohort. *Psychiatrica Fennica, 26*, 63–80.

Jones, P.B., Done, D.J. (1997). From birth to onset: a developmental perspective of schizophrenia in two national birth cohorts. In M.S. Keshavan, R.M. Murray (eds.), *Neurodevelopment and adult psychopathology* (pp. 119–136). Cambridge: Cambridge University Press.

Jones, P., Rodgers, B., Murray, R., Marmot, M. (1994). Child development risk factors for adult schizophrenia in the British 1946 birth cohort. *Lancet, 344(8934)*, 1398–1402.

Karlsson, J.L. (1984). Creative intelligence in relatives of mental patients. *Hereditas, 100*, 83–86

Karlsson, J.L. (2004). Psychosis and academic performance *British Journal of Psychiatry, 184*, 327–329.

Kendell, R.E., Gourlay, J. (1970). The clinical distinction between the affective psychoses and schizophrenia. *British Journal of Psychiatry, 117(538)*, 261–266.

Kendler, K.S., McGuire, M., Gruenberg, A.M., Walsh, D. (1994). Outcome and family study of the subtypes of schizophrenia in the west of Ireland. *American Journal of Psychiatry, 151(6)*, 849–856.

Kendler, K.S., Karkowski, L.M., Walsh, D. (1998). The structure of psychosis: latent class analysis of probands from the Roscommon Family Study. *Archives of General Psychiatry, 55(6)*, 492–499.

Kennedy, N., Everitt, B., Boydell, J., van Os, J., Jones, P.B., Murray, R.M. (2005a). Incidence and distribution of first-episode mania by age: results from a 35-year study. *Psychological Medicine, 35(6)*, 855–863.

Kennedy, N., Boydell, J., Kalidindi, S., Fearon, P., Jones, P.B., van Os, J., Murray, R.M. (2005b). Gender differences in incidence and age at onset of mania and bipolar disorder over a 35-year period in Camberwell, England. *American Journal of Psychiatry, 162(2)*, 257–262.

Kinney, D.K., Richards, R., Lowing, P.A., LeBlanc, D., Zimbalist, M.E., Harlan, P. (2001).

Creativity in offspring of schizophrenic and control parents: an adoption study. *Creativity Research Journal 13(1)*, 17–25.

Kirkbride, J.B., Fearon, P., Morgan, C., Dazzan, P., Morgan, K., Tarrant, J., Lloyd, T., Holloway, J., Hutchinson, G., Leff, J.P., Mallett, R.M., Harrison, G.L., Murray, R.M., Jones, P.B. (2006). Heterogeneity in incidence rates of schizophrenia and other psychotic syndromes: findings from the 3-center AeSOP study. *Archives of General Psychiatry, 63(3)*, 250–258.

Kirkpatrick, B., Buchanan, R.W., Ross, D.E., Carpenter, W.T.J. (2001). A separate disease within the syndrome of schizophrenia. *Archives of General Psychiatry, 58(2)*, 165–171.

Knutson, K.L., Turek, F.W. (2006). The U-shaped association between sleep and health: the 2 peaks do not mean the same thing. *Sleep, 29(7)*, 878–879.

Koenen, K.C., Moffitt, T.E., Roberts, A.L., Martin, L.T., Kubzansky, L., Harrington, H., Poulton, R., Caspis, A. (2009). Childhood IQ and adult mental disorders: a test of the cognitive reserve hypothesis. *American Journal of Psychiatry, 166*, 50–57

Krabbendam, L., van Os, J. (2005). Schizophrenia and urbanicity: a major environmental influence – conditional on genetic risk. *Schizophrenia Bulletin, 31(4)*, 795–799.

Krabbendam, L., Arts, B., van Os, J., Aleman, A. (2005). Cognitive functioning in patients with schizophrenia and bipolar disorder: a quantitative review. *Schizophrenia Research, 80(2–3)*, 137–149.

Kremen, W.S., Buka, S.L., Seidman, L.J., Goldstein, J.M., Koren, D., Tsuang, M.T. (1998). IQ decline during childhood and adult psychotic symptoms in a community sample: a 19-year longitudinal study. *American Journal of Psychiatry, 155(5)*, 672–677.

Kutcher, S., Robertson, H.A., Bird, D. (1998). Premorbid functioning in adolescent onset bipolar I disorder: a preliminary report from an ongoing study. *Journal of Affective Disorders, 51(2)*, 137–144.

Langholz, B., Clayton, D. (1994). Sampling strategies in nested case-control studies. *Environmental Health Perspectives, 102(Suppl 8)*, 47–51.

Last, J.M. (2001). *A dictionary of epidemiology*, 4th ed. Oxford: Oxford University Press.

Lawlor, D.A., Clark, H., Ronalds, G., Leon, D.A. (2006). Season of birth and childhood intelligence: findings from the Aberdeen Children of the 1950s cohort study. *British Journal of Educational Psychology, 76(Pt 3)*, 481–499.

Lee, C., McGlashan, T.H., Woods, S.W. (2005). Prevention of schizophrenia: can it be achieved? *CNS Drugs, 19(3)*, 193–206.

Li, D., Collier, D.A., He, L. (2006). Meta-analysis shows strong positive association of the neuregulin 1 (NRG1) gene with schizophrenia. *Human Molecular Genetics, 15(12)*, 1995–2002.

Lichtenstein, P., Bjork, C., Hultman, C.M., Scolnick, E., Sklar, P., Sullivan, P.F. (2006). Recurrence risks for schizophrenia in a Swedish national cohort. *Psychological Medicine, 36(10)*, 1417–1425.

Loomis, D., Richardson, D.B., Elliott, L. (2005). Poisson regression analysis of ungrouped data. *Occupational and Environmental Medicine, 62(5)*, 325–329.

Ludwig, A.M. (1992). Creative achievement and psychopathology: comparison among professions. *American Journal of Psychotherapy, 46(3)*, 330–356.

Ludwig, A.M. (1994). Mental illness and creative activity in female writers. *American Journal of Psychiatry, 151(11)*, 1650–1656.

Lundh, S. (2003). *National agency for education report no. 236: Descriptive data on childcare, schools and adult education in Sweden*. Stockholm: National Agency for Education, SE-106 20.

MacCabe, J.H., Aldouri, E., Fahy, T.A., Sham, P.C., Murray, R.M. (2002). Do schizophrenic patients who managed to get to university have a non-developmental form of illness? *Psychological Medicine, 32(3)*, 535–544.

MacCabe, J.H., Lambe, M.P., Cnattingius, S., Torrang, A., Bjork, C., Sham, P.C., David, A.S., Murray, R.M., Hultman, C.M. (2008). Scholastic achievement at age 16 and risk of schizophrenia and other psychoses: a national cohort study. *Psychological Medicine*, *38(8)*, 1133–1140.

MacCabe, J.H., Koupil, I., Leon, D.A. (2009). Lifetime reproductive output over two generations in patients with psychosis and their unaffected siblings: the Uppsala 1915–1929 Birth Cohort Multigenerational Study. *Psychological Medicine*, *39(10)*, 1667–1676.

MacCabe, J.H., Lambe, M.P., Cnattingius, S., Sham, P.C., David, A.S., Reichenberg, A., Murray, R.M., Hultman, C.M. (2010). Excellent school performance at age 16 and risk of adult bipolar disorder: a national cohort study. *British Journal of Psychiatry*, *196*, 109–115.

Makikyro, T., Isohanni, M., Moring, J., Oja, H., Hakko, H., Jones, P., Rantakallio, P. (1997). Is a child's risk of early onset schizophrenia increased in the highest social class? *Schizophrenia Research*, *23(3)*, 245–252.

Malaspina, D., Reichenberg, A., Weiser, M., Fennig, S., Davidson, M., Harlap, S., Wolitzky, R., Rabinowitz, J., Susser, E., Knobler, H.Y. (2005). Paternal age and intelligence: implications for age-related genomic changes in male germ cells. *Psychiatric Genetics*, *15(2)*, 117–125.

Mantel, N., Haenszel, W. (1959). Statistical aspects of the analysis of data from retrospective studies of disease. *Journal of the National Cancer Institute*, *22*, 719–748.

Marcelis, M., Navarro-Mateu, F., Murray, R., Selten, J.P., Van Os, J. (1998). Urbanization and psychosis: a study of 1942–1978 birth cohorts in The Netherlands. *Psychological Medicine*, *28(4)*, 871–879.

Mason, C.F. (1956). Pre-illness intelligence of mental hospital patients. *Journal of Consulting Psychology*, *20(4)*, 297–300.

Matte, T.D., Bresnahan, M., Begg, M.D., Susser, E. (2001). Influence of variation in birth weight within normal range and within sibships on IQ at age 7 years: cohort study. *British Medical Journal*, *323(7308)*, 310–314.

McGrath, J. (1999). Hypothesis: is low prenatal vitamin D a risk-modifying factor for schizophrenia? *Schizophrenia Research*, *40(3)*, 173–177.

McGrath, J.J. (2006). Variations in the incidence of schizophrenia: data versus dogma. *Schizophrenia Bulletin*, *32(1)*, 195–197.

McGrath, J., Scott, J. (2006). Urban birth and risk of schizophrenia: a worrying example of epidemiology where the data are stronger than the hypotheses. *Epidemiologia e Psichiatria Sociale*, *15(4)*, 243–246.

McGrath, J., Welham, J., Pemberton, M. (1995). Month of birth, hemisphere of birth and schizophrenia. *British Journal of Psychiatry*, *167(6)*, 783–785.

McGrath, J., Saha, S., Welham, J., El Saadi, O., MacCauley, C., Chant, D. (2004). A systematic review of the incidence of schizophrenia: the distribution of rates and the influence of sex, urbanicity, migrant status and methodology. *BMC Medicine*, *2*, 13.

McIntosh, A.M., Harrison, L.K., Forrester, K., Lawrie, S.M., Johnstone, E.C. (2005). Neuropsychological impairments in people with schizophrenia or bipolar disorder and their unaffected relatives. *British Journal of Psychiatry*, *186*, 378–385.

McNeil, T.F. (1971). Prebirth and postbirth influence on the relationship between creative ability and recorded mental illness. *Journal of Personality*, *39*, 391–406.

Morgan, C., Kirkbride, J., Leff, J., Craig, T., Hutchinson, G., McKenzie, K., Morgan, K., Dazzan, P., Doody, G.A., Jones, P., Murray, R., Fearon, P. (2007). Parental separation, loss and psychosis in different ethnic groups: a case-control study. *Psychological Medicine*, *37(4)*, 495–503.

Mortensen, P.B., Pedersen, C.B., Melbye, M., Mors, O., Ewald, H. (2003). Individual and familial risk factors for bipolar affective disorders in Denmark. *Archives of General Psychiatry*, *60(12)*, 1209–1215.

Mulvany, F., O'Callaghan, E., Takei, N., Byrne, M., Fearon, P., Larkin, C. (2001). Effect of social class at birth on risk and presentation of schizophrenia: case-control study. *British Medical Journal, 323(7326)*, 1398–1401.

Murphy, K.C., Jones, L.A., Owen, M.J. (1999). High rates of schizophrenia in adults with velo-cardio-facial syndrome. *Archives of General Psychiatry 56*, 940–945.

Murray, R.M., Lewis, S.W. (1987). Is schizophrenia a neurodevelopmental disorder? [editorial]. *British Medical Journal (Clinical Research Edition), 295(6600)*, 681–682.

Murray, R.M., Sham, P. van Os, J., Zanelli, J., Cannon, M., McDonald, C. (2004). A developmental model for similarities and dissimilarities between schizophrenia and bipolar disorder. *Schizophrenia Research, 71(2–3)*, 405–416.

Myhrman, A., Rantakallio, P., Isohanni, M., Jones, P., Partanen, U. (1996). Unwantedness of a pregnancy and schizophrenia in the child. *British Journal of Psychiatry, 169(5)*, 637–640.

Nasar, S. (1998). *A beautiful mind.* London: Faber and Faber.

Nelson, H.E. (1982). *The national adult reading test (NART).* Windsor: NFER-Nelson.

Nettle, D. (2001). *Strong imagination: madness, creativity and human nature.* Oxford: Oxford University Press.

Niklasson, A., Ericson, A., Fryer, J.G., Karlberg, J., Lawrence, C., Karlberg, P. (1991). An update of the Swedish reference standards for weight, length and head circumference at birth for given gestational age (1977–1981). *Acta Paediatrica Scandinavica, 80(8–9)*, 756–762.

Norio, R. (2003). Finnish disease heritage I: characteristics, causes, background. *Human Genetics, 112(5–6)*, 441–456.

Ogendahl, B.K., Agerbo, E., Byrne, M., Licht, R.W., Eaton, W.W., Mortensen, P.B. (2006). Indicators of fetal growth and bipolar disorder: a Danish national register-based study. *Psychological Medicine, 36(9)*, 1219–1224.

Öhman, B. (2005). *Multi-generation register 2004: a description of contents and quality.* Stockholm: Statistics Sweden.

Osler, M., Lawlor, D.A., Nordentoft, M. (2007). Cognitive function in childhood and early adulthood and hospital admission for schizophrenia and bipolar disorders in Danish men born in 1953. *Schizophrenia Research, 92(1–3)*, 132–141.

Owen, M.J., Craddock, N., O'Donovan, M.C. (2005). Schizophrenia: genes at last? *Trends in Genetics, 21(9)*, 518–525.

Pedersen, C.B., Mortensen, P.B. (2001). Family history, place and season of birth as risk factors for schizophrenia in Denmark: a replication and reanalysis. *British Journal of Psychiatry, 179*, 46–52.

Pedersen, C.B., Mortensen, P.B. (2006). Urbanicity during upbringing and bipolar affective disorders in Denmark. *Bipolar Disorders, 8(3)*, 242–247.

Perreira, K.M., Harris, K.M., Lee, D. (2006). Making it in America: high school completion by immigrant and native youth. *Demography, 43(3)*, 511–536.

Peters, E.R., Thornton, P., Siksou, L., Linney, Y., MacCabe, J.H. (2008). Specificity of the jump-to-conclusions bias in deluded patients. *British Journal of Clinical Psychology, 47(Pt 2)*, 239–244.

Popper K.R. (1983). *Realism and the aim of science. Postscript to the logic of scientific discovery,* vol I. Totawa, NJ: Rowan and Littlefield.

Rasanen, P., Tiihonen, J., Hakko, H. (1998). The incidence and onset-age of hospitalized bipolar affective disorder in Finland. *Journal of Affective Disorders, 48(1)*, 63–68.

Reichenberg, A., Weiser, M., Rabinowitz, J., Caspi, A., Schmeidler, J., Mark, M., Kaplan, Z., Davidson, M. (2002). A population-based cohort study of premorbid intellectual, language, and behavioral functioning in patients with schizophrenia, schizoaffective disorder, non-psychotic bipolar disorder. *American Journal of Psychiatry, 159(12)*, 2027–2035.

Reichenberg, A., Weiser, M., Rapp, M.A., Rabinowitz, J., Caspi, A., Schmeidler, J., Knobler,

H.Y., Lubin, G., Nahon, D., Harvey, P.D., Davidson, M. (2005). Elaboration on premorbid intellectual performance in schizophrenia: premorbid intellectual decline and risk for schizophrenia. *Archives of General Psychiatry, 62(12)*, 1297–1304.

Richards, M., Hardy, R., Kuh, D., Wadsworth, M.E. (2001). Birth weight and cognitive function in the British 1946 birth cohort: longitudinal population based study. *British Medical Journal, 322(7280)*, 199–203.

Richards, R., Kinney, D.K., Lunde, I., Benet, M., Merzel, A.P. (1988). Creativity in manic-depressives, cyclothymes, their normal relatives, and control subjects. *Journal of Abnormal Psychology, 97(3)*, 281–288.

Robin, N.H., Shprintzen, R.J. (2005). Defining the clinical spectrum of deletion 22q11.2. *Journal of Pediatrics, 147(1)*, 90–96.

Robinson, L.J., Thompson, J.M., Gallagher, P., Goswami, U., Young, A.H., Ferrier, I.N., Moore, P.B. (2006). A meta-analysis of cognitive deficits in euthymic patients with bipolar disorder. *Journal of Affective Disorders, 93(1–3)*, 105–115.

Schretlen, D.J., Buffington, A.L., Meyer, S.M., Pearlson, G.D. (2005). The use of word-reading to estimate "premorbid" ability in cognitive domains other than intelligence. *Journal of the International Neuropsychol Society, 11(6)*, 784–787.

Schwartz, S., Susser, E. (2006). The myth of the heritability index. In J.H. MacCabe, O. O'Daly, R.M. Murray, P. McGuffin, P. Wright (eds.), *Beyond nature and nurture in psychiatry: Genes, environment and their interplay* (pp. 19–26). Oxford: Informa Healthcare.

Scott, J., McNeill, Y., Cavanagh, J., Cannon, M., Murray, R. (2006). Exposure to obstetric complications and subsequent development of bipolar disorder: systematic review. *British Journal of Psychiatry, 189*, 3–11.

Seidman, L.J., Buka, S.L., Goldstein, J.M., Horton, N.J., Rieder, R.O., Tsuang, M.T. (2000). The relationship of prenatal and perinatal complications to cognitive functioning at age 7 in the New England Cohorts of the National Collaborative Perinatal Project. *Schizophrenia Bulletin, 26(2)*, 309–321.

Selten, J.P., van der Graaf, Y., van Duursen, R., Gispen-de Wied, C.C., Kahn, R.S. (1999). Psychotic illness after prenatal exposure to the 1953 Dutch Flood Disaster. *Schizophrenia Research, 35(3)*, 243–245.

Shprintzen, R.J. (2008). Velo-cardio-facial syndrome: 30 years of study. *Developmental Disabilities Research Reviews, 14(1)*, 3–10.

Sipos, A., Rasmussen, F., Harrison, G., Tynelius, P., Lewis, G., Leon, D.A., Gunnell, D. (2004). Paternal age and schizophrenia: a population based cohort study. *British Medical Journal, 329(7474)*, 1070.

Song, Y.M., Ha, M., Sung, J. (2007). Body mass index and mortality in middle-aged Korean women. *Annals of Epidemiology, 17(7)*, 556–563.

Srinivasan, T.N., Padmavati, R. (1997). Fertility and schizophrenia: evidence for increased fertility in the relatives of schizophrenic patients. *Acta Psychiatrica Scandinavica, 96(4)*, 260–264.

St Clair, D., Xu, M., Wang, P., Yu, Y., Fang, Y., Zhang, F., Zheng, X., Gu, N., Feng, G., Sham, P., He, L. (2005). Rates of adult schizophrenia following prenatal exposure to the Chinese famine of 1959–1961. *Journal of the American Medical Association, 294(5)*, 557–562.

STATA (2005). *Intercooled STATA 9.2 for Macintosh*. College Station, TX: Statacorp.

Statistical Analysis System Institute (SAS) (2006). *SAS 9.1.3 for UNIX*. Cary, NC: SAS Institute. (http://support.sas.com)

Statistiska Centralbyrån (2003). *Official Statistics of Sweden, 2003*. (www.scb.se)

StatTransfer (2005). Stat/Transfer 7 for Windows. Seattle, WA: Circle Systems.

Stefansson, H., Rujescu, D., Cichon, S., Pietiläinen, O.P., Ingason, A., Steinberg, S., *et al.*

(2008). Large recurrent micro-deletios associated with schizophrenia. *Nature, 455(7210),* 232–236.

Sternberg, R.J. (1998). *The triarchic mind: a new theory of human intelligence.* New York: Penguin.

Sternberg, R.J., Forsythe, G.B., Hedlund, J., Horvath, J.A., Wagner, R.K., Williams, W.M., Snook, S.A., Grigorenko, E.L. (2000). *Practical intelligence in everyday life.* New York: Cambridge University Press.

Stevenson, R.L. (1886). *Strange case of Dr Jekyll and Mr Hyde.* London: Longman's, Green and Co.

Strakowski, S.M., DelBello, M.P., Fleck, D.E., Adler, C.M., Anthenelli, R.M., Keck, P.E.J., Arnold, L.M., Amicone, J. (2007). Effects of co-occurring cannabis use disorders on the course of bipolar disorder after a first hospitalization for mania. *Archives of General Psychiatry, 64(1),* 57–64.

Swinnen, S.G., Selten, J.P. (2007). Mood disorders and migration: meta-analysis. *British Journal of Psychiatry, 190,* 6–10.

Tiihonen, J., Haukka, J., Henriksson, M., Cannon, M., Kieseppa, T., Laaksonen, I., Sinivuo, J., Lonnqvist, J. (2005). Premorbid intellectual functioning in bipolar disorder and schizophrenia: results from a cohort study of male conscripts. *American Journal of Psychiatry, 162(10),* 1904–1910.

Tohen, M., Calabrese, J.R., Sachs, G.S., Banov, M.D., Detke, H.C., Risser, R., Baker, R.W., Chou, J.C., Bowden, C.L. (2006). Randomized, placebo-controlled trial of olanzapine as maintenance therapy in patients with bipolar I disorder responding to acute treatment with olanzapine. *American Journal of Psychiatry, 163(2),* 247–256.

Torrey, E.F., Rawlings, R.R., Ennis, J.M., Merrill, D.D., Flores, D.S. (1996). Birth seasonality in bipolar disorder, schizophrenia, schizoaffective disorder and stillbirths. *Schizophrenia Research, 21(3),* 141–149.

Tracy, J.I., McGrory, A.C., Josiassen, R.C., Monaco, C.A. (1996). A comparison of reading and demographic-based estimates of premorbid intelligence in schizophrenia. *Schizophrenia Research, 22(2),* 103–109.

Tsuchiya, K.J., Agerbo, E., Byrne, M., Mortensen, P.B. (2004). Higher socio-economic status of parents may increase risk for bipolar disorder in the offspring. *Psychological Medicine, 34(5),* 787–793.

Vaittinen, P. (2003). *In-patient diseases in Sweden 1987–2001.* The National Board of Health and Welfare, Centre for Epidemiology. Stockholm: Official Statistics of Sweden.

van Os, J., Selten, J.P. (1998). Prenatal exposure to maternal stress and subsequent schizophrenia. The May 1940 invasion of The Netherlands [see comments]. *British Journal of Psychiatry, 172,* 324–326.

van Os, J., Jones, P., Lewis, G., Wadsworth, M., Murray, R. (1997). Developmental precursors of affective illness in a general population birth cohort. *Archives of General Psychiatry, 54(7),* 625–631.

van Os, J., Krabbendam, L., Myin-Germeys, I., Delespaul, P. (2005). The schizophrenia envirome. *Current Opinion in Psychiatry, 18(2),* 141–145.

Verdoux, H., Bourgeois, M. (1995). Social class in unipolar and bipolar probands and relatives. *Journal of Affective Disorders, 33(3),* 181–187.

Vernon, P.E. (1989). The nature–nuture problem in creativty. In J.A. Glover, R.R. Ronning, C.R. Reynolds (eds.), *Handbook of creativity* (pp. 93–110). New York: Plenum Press.

Waddell, C. (1998). Creativity and mental illness: is there a link? *Canadian Journal of Psychiatry, 43(2),* 166–172.

Walsh, B. (2003). Evolutionary quantitative genetics. In D.J. Balding, M. Bishop, C. Cannings (eds.), *Handbook of statistical genetics,* 2nd ed. (pp. 389–438). Chichester: John Wiley and Sons.

Walsh, T. McClellan, J.M., McCarthy, S.E., Addington, A.M., Pierce, S.B., Cooper, G.M., *et al.* (2008). Rare structural variants disrupt multiple genes in neurodevelopmental pathways in schizophrenia. *Science, 320(5875)*, 539–643.

Wechsler, D. (1997). *Wechsler Adult Intelligence Scale*, 3rd ed. London: Harcourt Brace and Company. Minnesota: The Psychological Corporation.

Weinberger, D.R. (1987). Implications of normal brain development for the pathogenesis of schizophrenia. *Archives of General Psychiatry, 44(7)*, 660–669.

Weiser, M., Reichenberg, A., Rabinowitz, J., Kaplan, Z., Mark, M., Nahon, D., Davidson, M. (2000). Gender differences in premorbid cognitive performance in a national cohort of schizophrenic patients. *Schizophrenia Research, 45(3)*, 185–190.

Wicks, S., Hjern, A., Gunnell, D., Lewis, G., Dalman, C. (2005). Social adversity in childhood and the risk of developing psychosis: a national cohort study. *American Journal of Psychiatry, 162(9)*, 1652–1657.

Williams, H.J., Owen, M.J., O'Donovan, M.C., (2007). Is COMT a susceptibility gene for schizophrenia. *Schizophrenia Bulletin, 33(3)*, 635.

Williams, N.M., O'Donovan, M.C., Owen, M.J. (2005). Is the dysbindin gene (DTNBP1) a susceptibility gene for schizophrenia? *Schizophrenia Bulletin, 31(4)*, 800–805.

World Health Organization (WHO) (1967). *International statistical classification of diseases and related health problems*, 8th ed. (ICD–8). Geneva: WHO.

World Health Organization (WHO) (1978). *International statistical classification of diseases and related health problems*, 9th ed. (ICD–9). Geneva: WHO.

World Health Organization (WHO) (1992). *International statistical classification of diseases and related health problems*, 10th ed. (ICD–10). Geneva: WHO.

Xu, B., Roos, J.L., Levy, S., van Rensburg, E.J., Gogos, J.A., Karayiorgon, M. (2008). Strong association of de novo copy number mutations with sporadic schizophrenia. *Nature Genetics, 40(7)*, 880–885.

Zammit, S., Allebeck, P., David, A.S., Dalman, C., Hemmingsson, T., Lundberg, I., Lewis, G. (2004). A longitudinal study of premorbid IQ score and risk of developing schizophrenia, bipolar disorder, severe depression, and other nonaffective psychoses. *Archives of General Psychiatry, 61(4)*, 354–360.

Index